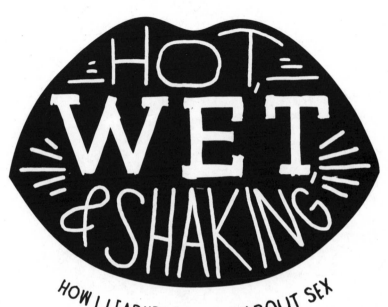

HOW I LEARNED TO TALK ABOUT SEX

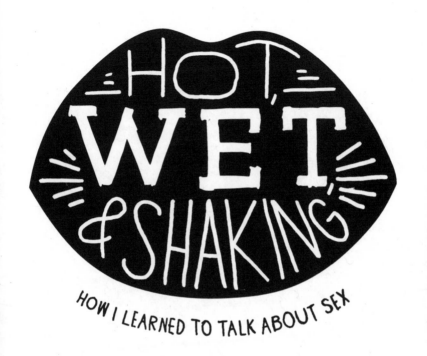

HOT, WET & SHAKING

HOW I LEARNED TO TALK ABOUT SEX

KALEIGH TRACE

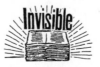

Invisible Publishing

Halifax & Toronto

Library and Archives Canada Cataloguing in Publication

Trace, Kaleigh, 1986-, author
    Hot, wet, and shaking : how I learned to
    talk about sex / Kaleigh Trace.

ISBN 978-1-926743-47-9 (pbk.)

    1. Trace, Kaleigh, 1986- --Sexual behavior. 2. Sex. 3. Women
with disabilities--Canada--Biography. 4. Feminists--Canada--
Biography. I. Title.

HV3013.T73A3 2014   362.4092 C2014-903616-7

Cover & Interior designed by Megan Fildes

Typeset in Laurentian and Slate by Megan Fildes
With thanks to type designer Rod McDonald

Printed and bound in Canada

Invisible Publishing
Halifax & Toronto
www.invisiblepublishing.com

We acknowledge the support of the Canada Council for the Arts, which last year
invested $157 million to bring the arts to Canadians throughout the country.

Invisible Publishing recognizes the support of the Province of Nova Scotia
through the Department of Communities, Culture & Heritage. We are pleased
to work in partnership with the Culture Division to develop and promote our
cultural resources for all Nova Scotians.

  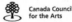 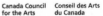

NOVA SCOTIA
Communities, Culture and Heritage

NOVA SCOTIA
NOUVELLE-ÉCOSSE

Canada Council   Conseil des Arts
for the Arts   du Canada

This book is dedicated to my younger self and all our younger selves. To those years we spent uncomfortably stumbling towards who we are. I am so grateful for all of the wrong turns I took that led me here.

What I have stumbled upon
has pleased me most.
— Eli Coppola

AN INTRODUCTION,
DEAR READER

Dear Reader,

Let me be honest.
I must confess:
I do not know what I am doing here.
I do not know where to start.
I am not sure that I am an expert. I am not sure that I am
an author. I am not sure I have a memoir in me, or anything
worth saying over the length of 200 pages.
I have never written a book before.

When I imagine people who write books, I imagine
Hemingway, hunting lions and then propping his feet
up on some chaise-longue like a boss and jamming out
a perfect piece of literature on his typewriter in a single
afternoon. Or I see Jeanette Winterson, falling in and out
of love and then moodily pouring her broken heart into
her work, constructing incredible sentences that make
a reader weep while sitting under the grey skies of Eng-
land. A writer looks like Leonard Cohen in a three piece
suit, passing poetry through his lips. It looks like Michael

Ondaatje, teaching us Toronto's history and immigrants' stories. It is Agatha Christie typing, typing, typing, in her upper class boudoir. It is Charles Bukowski fueling his brain and his books with booze.

I am not these things. I am messier than all of that and this town is more mundane. There are no lions here. I am not wearing a suit, just yesterday's underwear and stained jeans. I am not smoking a cigarette nor drinking a glass of wine. When I get drunk I just fall over, and sometimes even pee my pants a little. Smoking irritates my asthma. On my desk are only this laptop and a yogurt container grown mouldy, a few coffee cups with last week's dregs and a small bundle of lint and gum wrappers pulled out from my coat pocket. There are no windows in this room. And it smells weird too.

These credentials, full of everyday details and lacking entirely in romance, make me feel nervous and ill-equipped. This space does not feel perfect enough to write a book in. My life experiences do not seem exciting enough to narrate. My underwear are too dirty. My hair is a mess.

However, I should start somewhere. And despite all of my aforementioned uncertainty, there are some things that I do know for sure.

Let me begin with these:

1. I AM A (TOUGH AS FUCK) WOMAN WITH A DISABILITY.

And I have been for nearly as long as I can remember. In 1995, my family and I were in a car accident. This accident caused me to sustain a severe spinal cord injury. Doctors diagnosed me as having paraplegia, and I spent a part of my childhood in a wheelchair. However, children's bodies, with all of their youthful will, are capable of incredible feats. I was out of my wheelchair within a year, stumbling and slipping and fighting to keep up with all the other kids. Today, I amble around with a serious swagger. It looks a little like I am always dancing. My wobbly two-step gets me to all of the places that I need to go: upstairs, downstairs and across long distances. I am *in love* with my body: the way my thighs scissor in and out, the way my feet curl and tumble in on one another, the broad width of my shoulders that support me when I trip and fall.

Having this beautiful, disabled body and living in this world with such an obvious difference has shaped me irreversibly. Being disabled informs every single experience I have with every person, every street corner, every building and every set of stairs. I am, and have always been, constantly reminded that my body is different from "normal" bodies, that it is actually physically impossible for me to conform to hegemonic standards of being. I can't fit in because my legs won't let me. My shattered spinal cord bars me from regularity.

I cannot walk through city streets without being disabled, and so I cannot write a book without being the same. This book will not be about my "perseverance," "courage," and/or "bravery." Those words have never felt like friends, with their implicit condescension. Instead, this book will be about who I am, in my entirety. I am a woman, I am disabled, and I am an avid eater of eggs, to name only a few. These identities overlap and move in and out of one another, criss-crossing and informing me and my universe. I cannot *not* talk about them. I cannot *not* write about them.

2. I AM A SEX-POSITIVE SEX EDUCATOR.

Sex, sex, sex. It is kind of my deal. What this looks like: I teach blow job workshops. Seriously. I am a blow job master, an expert, the top of the top. Once a month I wave around a big, silicone cock in front of a group of people and I get paid to have this much fun.

But, of course, that is oversimplifying it. I suppose that on the surface being a blow job expert sounds like a pretty specific skill, one that would perhaps not be applicable outside of my current work environment (I work at a sex shop). You may think this job title and skill set make me seem vulgar (I may be). You may think that this book is not for you. And I guess it may not be, especially if you are my family member and reading a book about my sex life makes you wildly uncomfortable (understandable, and in which case: stop now! Close the cover and put down these pages!). But, really, this book could be just the thing for you. And really, so could blow job classes. Because being a sex-positive, feminist sex educator is not really about blow jobs at all. I was just being facetious.

When I teach those classes, when I go to the shop and talk about sex all day long, when I write a blog post about sex, I am not only talking about the practicalities of doing it. I am not necessarily talking about how much fun sex is, though sometimes I am. I am not necessarily being explicit, though sometimes I am doing that too. Instead, what I am trying to do when I go on and on and on about sex is subvert those boring, repressive ideas that we are taught about the fine act of fucking.

Talking about sex is important because we live in a world that is saturated with it. Sex is absolutely everywhere. It is on the sidebar of the website you are looking at. It is on the billboards lining our city streets. It is on commercial breaks and in plot lines. It is the climax, the end goal, the outcome, the problem, and the solution. And, despite its constant and inescapable presence, the image of sex that we are force fed is both boring and exclusive.

If I were to believe everything I see, then I would believe that sex only happens between thin people. Only men with abdominal muscles do it. Only women with big tits get to bang. Men and women only do it with each other. Sex is for straight people, and sex only ever happens between two of them, never more or fewer than that. Sex is for white people. Sex is for pretty people. Sex is for able-bodied young people. Sex is spontaneous. Sex involves penetration. Sex lasts approximately 4.2 minutes. Sex happens in bedrooms, at night. Sex is predictable.

How very, deeply boring. What these insidious images of sex leave out are some of the best parts. What we are not hearing about is how sex can be kinky and subversive and very, very naughty in such fun and consensual ways. We are not seeing people of size get down. We are not seeing people with disabilities doin' it on the regular, not in their chairs nor in their beds. In mainstream media, we rarely see sexy images of people of colour that don't posit them as some exotified other. Nor do we see fair and equitable depictions of women's bodies, in all of their curvaceous beauty, experiencing pleasure. We don't see men's bodies being anything other than sexually dominant and capable and sure of themselves. We do not see bodies that refuse to conform to this restrictive gender binary. And we do not get to see that sex can be weird and awkward either. We do not see sex where someone accidentally farts. Poop and pee never happen in intimate moments. That moment when we realize that the position we are in does not work, where we get stuck with our legs above our heads, where we trip and fall or gag or barf or stumble or put things in the wrong places: those are all cut out and photo-shopped, removed from our sensible realities.

But sex does not work that way. Sex is weird, and wonderful, and dirty, and awkward, and kinky, and queer, and can consensually happen between all sorts of people, anywhere, at any time of day. That is the real life reality of this act with which we as a society are so preoccupied.

As a sex-positive, feminist sex educator, I find myself talking about the realities of real life sex all the time. And what I have found is that people think it is really embarrassing. Nobody seems to want to talk about the intricate and human and silly things that happen when we try to stick our bodies together. And so, in response, I talk louder and louder and louder and LOUDER. My mouth gets more filthy. I try to push boundaries even further. I want to be even bolder, because I believe that this shaming silence that surrounds our collective sex lives is what leads to us all having bad sex. It is why we judge other people's sexuality. It is why we don't know how to respect one another's bodies and one another's boundaries. It is why we don't know what consent can look like, and why sexual assault and rape can happen. It is why homophobia persists and why transphobia exists.

I am not arguing that just by openly discussing pussy farts, cum shots, and butt plugs, the world will be a better place, no one will be hurt, and we will all live in a blissful utopia where enthusiastic, consenting orgies abound and we each orgasm every time. That would be unrealistic. However, I do believe that the more and more we talk about that which we have such a hard time talking about, then we will all feel a little less ashamed and we will all be a little more open to new possibilities and new kinds of pleasure. And sex will come to mean something more than putting a penis in a vagina. And beauty will become something more than being able-bodied, young and white. And sexual autonomy and expression will be something that we will all have the right to. And consent will evolve into something that we will all be versed in practicing. It is on account of these hopes that I talk about sex all of the time. Loudly. On principle.

What this means is that I cannot write a book without writing about sex. And I cannot write about sex without writing about all of the ways that it is funny, uncouth, and weird.

3. IT BEGAN AS A BLOG AND NOW IT IS THIS BOOK(!)

Eventually, talking about sex at work every day was not enough. Conversations with customers would begin, thoughts would be provoked, and then they would walk out of the store happy, sex toy in hand. I would be left standing there with my mind whirling and wanting more. It felt like I was engaging in unsatisfactory sex with this whole city: the kind of sex where people tell me what they want, I give them what they need, and then it is over before I've finished. And so, rather than going home and masturbating, as one is left to do after having unsatisfactory sex, I began going home to write.

At work my brain would get turned on. The conversations I had with customers would get me thinking about sex, feminism, gender identity, sexual fluidity, patriarchy, and all of that shit which affects our relationships to our bodies. Rather than work out all of my questions with unsuspecting clients who are really just trying to make a simple transaction, I would go home and pour my throbbing thoughts out into my computer. I would write it all down until I was satiated.

So began my blog, *The Fucking Facts*, and so here I am now. Within a year, that blog led to this book deal. Now I sit here slightly daunted, trying to amass all my well-lubricated ideas about sex into a single, cohesive volume. Something that will make some sense. Something that will mean a thing or two to someone. Something that will glue together all the mixed-up and jumbled, strong and unwavering, new and exciting ideas that I have about sex and feminism and disability into a single pretty and powerful printed piece. I am still unsure of all of the versions of myself and where exactly I fit in this world of identities. I am still working out how I got here and where I even began. I am entirely clueless as to where this is all going. But here's hoping that in the following stories, we sort a few things out.

I may be doing this all backwards. I imagine that most people have a book idea, they take that fresh and new idea to a publisher, and that publisher then helps them deliver. Instead, I had a blog and then a publisher told me that I was pregnant with a book. Now it is all on me to push this book out of my vagina. Or out from my fingers. Or maybe my brain? Wherever it is that books come from (I wish it were a stork).

So, let me both conclude and begin it all by saying:

This is my first try.

Be gentle on me.

I will try to be honest.

I will try to be kind.

I will definitely be dirty (in the best way).

A BAG OF DICKS

Something happens to you when you begin working at sex shop. When sex becomes your bread and butter, it is entirely possible to forget that for some people, this topic is still taboo. Your boundaries change, your sense of "normalcy" is forever altered. Things happen to you that you thought would never happen: you find yourself explaining queer sex to your grandmother; you will casually and without consideration discuss the healing power of orgasms with a stranger on the bus. You descend, with only some discomfort, into the realm of being considered a total weirdo. And eventually it becomes more comfortable there in Weirdodom, a place where you no longer have to conform to obligatory social norms. However, arriving at that point may involve some...bumps.

I am running late. I am almost always running late, which I believe is one of the inevitabilities of being a classic, type-A, overworked overachiever. I am running late and I am multi-tasking. Also inevitable. If you are a person who wants to do everything, you must eventually learn to do everything simultaneously. Things will get done faster if you do them all at once. Or at least this is the theory that I am currently putting to some rigorous practical testing. It is for the good of science that I am maintaining a phone conversation while buying groceries, rushing to work, and double-checking my day planner to ascertain what exactly I am doing later and where I am going. This is all an experiment to improve my efficiency.

I would put the phone down if I could. Talking on the phone while in line at the grocery store is, I believe, the epitome of being an entitled asshole. As if the person ringing me through is not really human and therefore does not deserve my full attention. As if the people behind me in line really give a shit about my one side of this unnecessary conversation I am forcing them to listen to. But right now this phone call is inescapable. I said I was "maintaining a conversation," but really I am just repeatedly muttering "mmm." I can't interject much anyway. It is my most neurotic friend Jason on the other end, and cutting him off now would be tantamount to leaving the toilet paper roll empty, or not filling the stapler, or letting food accumulate in the catcher of the kitchen sink. It would be one of those little things with the capacity to annoy him so thoroughly that it is best to just avoid the act entirely. He is in the middle of giving me a remarkably detailed account of his second date with the woman he has been trying to seduce for months, and I recognize that it is crucial for him to see this narrative through in order to alleviate some of his anxiety. Is it a sign that she said she, "loved his cooking"? Should he text her today or wait two days to avoid seeming too eager? Is there a subtext to the fact that she told him her nail polish colour was called "Killer Flirt"?! I am not expected to answer any of these questions. He just needs to ask them aloud. So despite my social sensibilities, I continue this phone conversation for Jason's benefit. I mumble my "mmm-hmms" and "ohs" and general reassurances while I conduct my daily business.

On the plus side, I look good today. I took the time to brush my teeth and put on deodorant this morning. I am teaching a fellatio workshop tonight and so I am trying to pass as an adult woman who knows what she is doing. And while for the most part I do (know what I am doing, that is), I do not always look that way, when my hair is matted and my T-shirt is on backwards. But today is different. My teeth are clean, and my hair is brushed. I have lipstick on and it has not yet (I hope) smudged its way onto my pearly whites. I am a woman. I am a blow job expert. I am in control.

Except that I cannot find my wallet, and I just dropped my keys on the ground, and the teen boy cashier is looking at me impatiently as I scramble to pay him and get out of the way. The woman with her baby in line behind me is also glaring at me, disgruntled and annoyed. I am holding up everybody's day. I wish I could hang up my fucking cell phone already.

And that is when it happens. I am standing in line, with what feels like 100 frustrated people queued up behind me, with a bored teenager watching me and waiting, and I pull out a big, white, gleaming, silicone dick. What I think is my wallet is in fact my tool for tonight's workshop. A nice clean dildo, fresh and ready for me to display. Later, I will use this cock to teach anatomy and techniques. Later, it will be appropriate for me to be holding a dick in my hand, because people will have paid for that, and will have come expecting me to do that very thing. But now I am here, in line at an over-priced grocery store wielding a giant dick while a bunch of upper-class, middle-aged women stare at me, shocked. The baby begins to cry, not realistically because I have stolen his innocence, but it does feel that way.

"It's for work," I say by way of explanation. As though having a dildo in one's bag for work is entirely common. On the other side of my phone I hear Jason grumble "You're not listening to me, are you?" In front of me, the cashier continues to stare at me with his mouth ajar and his braces gleaming. I shove the cock back in my bag, find my wallet, grab my groceries, and flee.

This is not a lone experience. Things like this are always happening to me. It seems as though I always have vibrators and condoms, lube and butt plugs pouring from my pockets and bulging out of my bag. Just earlier this week I was caught by a truck driver with one hand down my pants as I frantically drove in circles looking for parking. There was a reasonable explanation for this. I was not just jerking it on my commute to work. I had just short-sightedly decided to test out a clitoral stimulating gel earlier that morning. I had assumed it would do nothing, that its "herbal, aphrodisiac ingredients" were bullshit buzz words that would not really get my clit hard nor my juices flowing. I dripped the tingling liquid onto my stuff, threw my pants on, and headed out the door. Unfortunately, the bottle was true to its word. The tingle set in while I was in the car, halfway to work. But rather then turn me on with its "gentle warmth," it started to burn and burn and burn. It felt like my clitoris was dangerously engorged, like it might actually fall off and I would find a little fleshy nub jamming around down by my brake pedal later. Frantically, I shoved my hands down my pants and started rubbing, hoping to absorb the gel onto my fingers and free my junk from its fiery grasp. That is when the truck driver just happened to look down into my car from his high-up perch in the neighbouring lane—while I was furiously rubbing myself just like any other car-driving pervert.

I have found myself thoughtlessly reading *A Hand in the Bush: The Fine Art of Vaginal Fisting* on the bus, beside a probably quite nice and now deeply disturbed eighty-year-old gentleman. I have detailed my sexual exploits to my co-worker in a booth at a small family restaurant, forgetting that not everyone talks about ejaculating while they shove mayonnaise and french fries into their mouths. I have showed my dick to a grocery store clerk and have had a truck driver watch me rub my cunt. By now, these experiences are comfortably predictable. My sense of propriety was a work-related casualty that has long been dead and buried.

AND THE WARMTH
SPREAD OVER US

When considering my early sexual experiences, it makes so much sense that I have wound up in the work that I am in. My interest in talking about sex is most certainly linked to the fact that for a long time I was very, very bad at having it. Really. I am not just being modest. I may be something of a pseudo sex expert now, but it has not always been this way. I have, in fact, committed what one would think are remarkably obvious sexual faux pas throughout the span of my relatively short life thus far. And I refuse to believe that all of my slip ups, mishaps, and total mistakes are my fault alone. No—I blame society. (I'm not joking).

Like many of you, I was once a teenager. If you remember being a teenager, than you remember that it is a truly awful experience. It is a time in your life that is full of regrettable outfits, actions, and hair decisions. You are riddled with near-constant emotional turmoil and ever-present skin problems. You can't really figure out who you are, what you want, or where you are going. And, you smell weird. Or at least this is how it was for me. I hated being a teenager.

As a teen, I was subject to all of the aforementioned universal teen experiences: the hair, the hormones, the smells.

On top of that, though, I had this whole disability thing to grapple with. I was doubly confused. All of the already mystifying adolescent changes were accentuated by the stark reality that my body was like no one else's. I did not know one single disabled person, other than myself. Based on my rural Ontario context, there was no one in the known universe like me. Given that I was a human anomaly, I could not figure out what the fuck my body was doing, nor how it was going to overcome the trials of teenhood. Both my present and my future seemed bleak.

The options for my post-high school, adult future, as presented to me by my immediate surroundings, were fairly homogenous. If I were to follow the trajectory of most people I knew, I would have done one of two options. Option One: marry, help my husband on the farm, and reproduce. Option Two: go to university in the nearest city, marry, help my husband on the farm, and reproduce. Neither One nor Two enticed me much. I could not imagine myself fitting into that framework. Try lifting hay bales with a limp. Try milking cows with chronic back pain. It sounded less than ideal. Plus, I've never liked cows. However, the thing that did entice me was adulthood. I wanted out of high school, out of my small town, and out of puberty. Desperately. So while these fairly normative narratives of what being an adult could look like were unappealing to me, I wanted to discover it nonetheless. And I wanted something different.

This is when I became obsessed with the idea of having sex. All I wanted to do was It. While this is probably a common enough adolescent sentiment, my preoccupation came from a different, more convoluted angle. I was not particularly interested in the act itself. I did not want to have sex to satiate all of my raging teen hormones. It was not that I could not stop thinking about it, nor that I thought it would necessarily feel good. I had never been overcome by any insatiable, physical, lusty urges. I had never even masturbated before. No, I wanted to do it for other reasons. I wanted to have sex because I believed it was my ticket into adulthood. I thought it would give me some answers. Sex was just a means to an end. The end, in my mind, was becoming a woman.

This all makes some sense really, as complicated as it may sound. I was a teenager in a town that barely knew what the internet was. Okay, many people knew what it was, but it was pretty hard to get, considering we lived amongst the endless, golden corn crops of Absolutely Nowhere. Attempts to access the so-called "Information Super Highway" began with the laborious, high-pitched beeps and squeals of the internet dialing up, and ended with any incoming phone call. Needless to say, I had very little access to radical ideas, to different ways of being, or to any information about sex. Sex was a total mystery to me, something that adults did in big cities like New York or Toronto. Sure, some of my girlfriends were having it with older boys in neighbouring towns, but to me this didn't sound like "real sex." My friend's descriptions of fumbling around in the backseat of their parents' car sounded more like cumbersome wrestling. I wanted to have what I believed was the sophisticated, true-to-life adult sex that happened in movies. I wanted to be admitted into the secret society of "real womanhood."

While I wanted to have sex with all of my being, I was simultaneously terrified of doing it. No one had ever explained to me how it really worked, and so I was not entirely sure what the act consisted of. I knew the basics. I understood that a penis went in a vagina. But I assumed there was more to it than just that. I imagined that both parties involved in the act had to move around a lot. I imagined a lot of bending over, leg-lifting, and a series of rapid pelvic thrusts. I could not do any of these things. My disability meant that my motion below the waist was pretty compromised, as was my sensation. I was not able to feel things that happened below my hipbones the way that an able-bodied person could. I wondered if I would I even be able to tell if a penis was in my vagina. And then that question led me to wondering if my vagina was supposed to do something once the penis was in it? Did other people's vaginas do something? Because mine seemed to just sit there.

These were pretty intimate questions, questions that I was too embarrassed to share with anyone. And these unanswered questions made me really anxious. I held a deep, dark fear that maybe I wouldn't be able to have sex at all. That maybe I would fail at this act and that failure would leave me trapped in what I believed to be the most boring adulthood available. What if my vaginal (mis)behaviour confined me to live in a small town forever?! Considering that such an outcome seemed to me like a fate worse than death, I decided to face my fears and do it—I would try to fuck. The only way to get some answers was to risk it.

Enter Dan. He was my first real boyfriend. I set about dating him out of neither lust nor love, but my obsessive adulthood-attaining endeavour. He would be The One, I decided. He met all of my required credentials. For one, he was a boy. For two, he was my boyfriend. For three, he wanted to have sex with me. That was really all I needed. I was so determined to do it that I was not going to set the bar too high. And of course, Dan was a nice enough dude. He loved me, he had a truck, and he had really great hair. We talked on the phone after school every night and spent our lunch hours making out down by the quarry, just off school property. Our relationship felt like a perfect pathway to meeting my goals. After eight months of us going steady, I decided it was time.

I, of course, undertook some initial preparations to ready myself for the act. While for most of my peers this would have meant bashfully buying a box of condoms at the gas station in the next town over, my planning strategy was more involved. The first step was to develop a series of rigorous exercises which I would perform every night before falling asleep. I would lie in my bed and furtively contort my body into awkward positions. First, I would lift my butt high off the mattress, thrusting my pelvis into the air. In that half-raised state I would then struggle to spread my legs as wide apart as possible, using my arms to shuffle my knees outward. Wary of the way that this stance created a triple chin, I would attempt to perform this workout while all the while looking lascivious. My eyebrows would be provocatively arched. I would open my lips in a way that, I hoped, looked sensual. Should my ankles give out or my knees buckle I would resolutely try and try again. I believed that these poses were critical to having sex and I practiced them as a crucial preemptive practice to fucking. I was a dedicated exerciser.

The second preparatory act was to enlist the help of a more experienced sex guide. Those deep, dark questions—like what my vagina was supposed to do—were too tender to ask of anyone. But I felt I should at least seek out some more general advice. I enrolled Katherine for the job. Katherine was not only a good friend but one of the most sexually active people I knew. Our teen years had looked very different thus far, which is to say that unlike myself, Katherine was a girl who grew up fast. While I had passed my summers pumping gas at the local gas station (AKA sitting on a lawn chair), she had spent all of hers away at summer camp. From June through July, Katherine's parents would send her off to different parts of the province, ostensibly to learn such skills as kayaking and wilderness training. Unbeknownst to them, Katherine would instead acquire much more incendiary life lessons. She had come back from her various summer excursions with hickeys, nipple piercings, and sordid stories of which I had never before heard the like. Considering that thus far my forays around the bases had not gotten me much farther than first, I knew she could teach me a thing or two. We scheduled a Friday night "study session" to be held in the privacy of her bedroom.

Katherine had obviously done this before. I arrived at her house to find her prepared with plenty of fruit, pilfered from her parents' kitchen: bananas, cucumbers, carrots, peaches, melons, and plums. She knew just which produce best suited sex tutorials.

The fruit, my anatomical guides, lay lined up across her black satin bedspread. I sat on the floor opposite the bed, ready to learn. This had been the bedroom where I had first gotten my period a year prior, where I had first kissed a boy, and where I had learned to put on makeup. Katherine's room had become the de facto location for rites of passage.

"Here," Katherine said, passing me a Smirnoff Ice cooler (her favourite drink).

I cracked open the bottle and gulped.

She stood beside the bed looking like a professional. A cigarette dangled from her hot pink lips and her La Senza push-up miracle bra was achieving its desired effect. À la Britney Spears, the waist band of her thong peeked out above her low-rise jeans. With one hand on her hips she launched into her lesson.

"You're not hopeless, but you do have a lot to learn," she began. "Let's start with this." She picked up the banana. "This is a dick." Next she took a bite out of the plum, and with her mouth full, she held up the soft, exposed inner pulp and explained, "this is a vagina."

Katherine proved to be an immersive instructor. Her food-based lesson in human sexuality went on for well over an hour. She extrapolated on everything from how to properly shape one's lips around a banana/dick, to how to avoid "pussy farts" (something I had never even heard of, let alone thought to avoid). I sat through it all enraptured, getting progressively drunk on Smirnoff coolers. Nearly everything that Katherine talked about was a revelation to me. By the time she was through, I was overwhelmed and even more scared. Learning that I knew nothing made sex seem all the more daunting.

But I could not back out now. Dan and I had set a date and I was not going to cancel it. Everything was in place. His dad was going to be away for the weekend and my parents thought I would be staying at a friend's. I had been practicing my exercises for months and I felt as physically ready as I'd ever be. Plus, Katherine had gifted me a congratulatory box of condoms. The time was now.

The following Friday night found me in Dan's bedroom. We sat facing each other on his bed. We were both naked except for our underwear, me in a sports bra and what I considered to be my sexiest pair of panties (pink with a cartoon cat on the front) and he in tattered boxer briefs. Neither one of us would look directly at the other. I focused my eyes on the glowing light of the candles I had spread around the room and tried to remember everything Katherine had taught me. Dan fiddled with the box of condoms, tossing it from one hand to the other.

"So, this is gonna be fun," he said, and nodded at me reassuringly.

"Uh, yeah," I said frowning.

"You ready?" he asked.

"Yeah," I said and started kissing him.

Kissing was familiar. I began to calm down. "I got this," I thought. I began to calm down and hoped that everything would be totally intuitive. We made out for a while, our skinny arms fumbling around one another's skinny bodies, our hands hesitantly groping at each other. When I felt Dan's hard-on press up against my thigh, I pulled his boxers down like I knew what I was doing. My hands felt for his penis. I had always kept my eyes closed while kissing because I thought that was the appropriately adult thing to do. But now I opened them, wanting to see it. I peeked down and immediately stopped kissing him. Dan's junk was much more intimidating than Katherine's banana had been. I pulled away.

"Don't be scared," he offered kindly. "Just pretend it's a Mars Bar."

I took a deep breath. And unfortunately, I took Dan's attempt at a reassuring metaphor literally. I bent down, put my mouth around his penis, and bit it. Perhaps it was all the food employed in my first-ever sex tutorial. Or maybe it was the performance anxiety making me do strange things. Either way, when I began my first attempt at sex, I began it with my teeth. What I had hoped would be a preliminary blow job turned into a hard-earned lesson of What Not To Do. As my teeth sank into his skin, Dan yelped with fear and pain. I quickly unclenched my jaw and recoiled. We both jumped up, pulled our clothes on, and proceeded to not look directly at each other. I don't think we ever looked directly at each other again. We went to sleep that night without having sex and without ever really talking about it. We broke up a week later.

It follows that the remainder of my high school career remained predominantly sex-less. That fairly traumatizing experience with Dan kept me off the saddle for quite a while. I did, however, eventually have penetrative sex and when it happened, it happened without teeth or fanfare. In fact, it happened in exactly the way I could have predicted it would if I had not spent so much time worrying about it.

It was at a barn party celebrating our high school graduation. After enough drinks had been consumed, I unceremoniously angled myself into the backseat of my station wagon with a boy I had known since I was five. We proceeded to engage in the predictably uncomfortable paired aerobic activities that we classified as sex. It was unclear if my years of late-night exercises had made the experience any better, or at the very least not totally terrible. Either way, in the end, the thing that I had spent so much time planning for lasted roughly five minutes and did absolutely nothing in the way of making me feel like a woman. It was remarkable only in that it was so unremarkable.

By the time I finally got around to doing It, I had already gotten a scholarship to a far off university, anyway. I had ceased framing sex as some sort of Escape from Small Town strategy and I was no longer as preoccupied with attaining adulthood. My disability related worries not withstanding, I fucked in my backseat that night just to prove to myself that I could. Knowing at least that much, I left town shortly thereafter and never moved back.

From rural Ontario, I resettled myself in Halifax, both to pursue post-secondary education and to continue my bumbling forays in strange men's nether regions. As one may imagine, my one night stand—with a boy I had spent my childhood eating sand with—had not given me many reassurances. All I had learned thus far about sex was to not bite a penis, but other than that I was uncertain about most everything. I knew I could at the very least do it in some capacity, but my deep, dark anxieties persisted. The role of my vagina continued to be enigmatic. The type of mobility sex required was still an unknown variable. I still wanted answers. So I continued to try and learn through trial by fire.

I met Matthew within two months of having moved to Halifax. This was back when you could still smoke inside bars and you could easily doctor an ID with a drop of black nail polish. My eighteen years of age now reading as twenty-eight, I slipped in and out of downtown bars unnoticed. Matthew and I met at a club called The Attic, previously known as My Apartment, later known as The Dome. He caught me as I stumbled around the dance floor in high-heeled boots I should never have tried to wear. There I was again—acting out an unconvincing performance as an able-bodied adult woman. I am hopeless in heels. Matthew grabbed my arm and rebalanced me as I tottered and teetered and tail-spinned out of an ungraceful dance maneuver. I looked up to thank my leaning post and saw that he was tall and handsome. Very, very tall, actually. So tall that I gave up trying to verbally communicate anything to him in the crowded bar. We wordlessly danced for a while, or rather, he held me up as we swayed back and forth, standing close together. At the end of the night, I gave him my number, feeling sheepish. Considering that all cultural commentary likens one's competency on the dance floor to their skills in the bedroom, I felt I had just given a rather unimpressive first impression. It was clear to Matthew that I could not cut a rug. If I couldn't dance, could I fuck? And would a very tall, handsome man even want to fuck me? My high school sexual history had not followed me across the country, but the damage it had done to my self-confidence had.

Luckily, Matthew could not tell from dancing with me that I had only had sex once in the back of my car for five minutes. He called me the next day and we went on our first date shortly thereafter.

I would describe Matthew and our preliminary dates if I could, but other than his towering height, I can barely remember anything about him or our time together before the incident. The lone characteristic that remains to mark my memories of that guy is his incessant need to perform renditions of Dave Chappelle skits. Matthew loved Dave Chappelle. He could recite nearly the entire script of *Half Baked* and would gladly do so at any time.

It is entirely possible that I don't recall our first few chaste dates because they were mostly composed of me listening to the tired repetition of marijuana-related jokes. Needless to say, it wasn't love. But Matthew had other things I was interested in. Specifically, he was older than me and he had his own apartment. I believed that these credentials could indicate that with Matthew I just may experience the sophisticated, adult sex I had once imagined. I ambitiously hoped that with him I would figure out what exactly sex was *really* meant to look like and whether or not I would be physically able to do it. Despite all of my sexual anxieties and past mortifications, I was still so wildly curious that I wasn't going to entirely give up on fucking just yet.

It was our third or maybe our fourth date when he invited me over under the pretext of watching *The Chappelle Show*. Watching TV together is always a pretext. So we acted out each of those predetermined gestures of what happens when two people who really just want to have sex watch TV together: we sat too close together on the couch, our hands inched across the worn fabric towards one another, our arms wrapped around each other, and then eventually we were in a horizontal two-person pile-up.

I knew right away that I had to pee. This is because a) as a general rule I always have to pee; and b) in situations that intimidate me that near-constant urge is multiplied by ten. It was no surprise when I felt that telltale tingle in my groins. Typically a part of being disabled for me is the constant responsibility of what the medical industry refers to as "bladder management." What this means: my bladder, unlike the bladder of some others, does its own thing and all I have to do is manage it. It pees when it wants to, whether or not I myself have signaled that it is an appropriate time to let loose. In the past it has decided to empty itself while I was talking to my first big crush, while I was kayaking in the ocean and while I was on an airplane, stuck in my seat during takeoff. Having such a domineering bladder is pretty inconvenient, and so to better control it, I starve it. Liquid intake is kept to a minimum before and during dates, movies, plane rides, and any other situation where toilets are not at the ready. Catheterization[1] must also happen pretty often, just to make

---

1. Catheterization is something that a lot of people do. A catheter is a clear, plastic tube-y thing that is inserted into the urethra and reaches up into the bladder. Some people have a catheter inserted all the time while others, like myself, do intermittent self-catheterization. This means that when I feel the need to pee I stick the tube-y thing into my urethra and pee comes out. I use a 14 French catheter, which you don't really need to know, but it sounds kind of sexy.

sure that my bladder is sufficiently empty and cannot surprise attack my jeans (and my sense of pride) at inopportune moments. All this to say that I should have been much more attentive to the tingle.

But I wasn't. I just did not want to be. At the age of eighteen I was still painfully aware of the ways in which I wasn't "normal." My overactive bladder was very far from normal. I had been counting and I had already excused myself and run to the bathroom three times on this date thus far. I felt that this number of bathroom breaks was clearly bizarre. I was sure that this handsome, older man would be completely turned off by my excessive bodily functions. I was even willing to bet that one more pee break would end this date and cancel the sweet sex I was expecting. My only option: hold it.

We moved off the couch and progressed into his bedroom. All the while my knees were shaking with the effort to control my bladder. He pressed me up against the wall and kissed my neck. It may have felt good but I was too distracted to notice. My shirt came off and next his belt. He threw me on the bed. We continued to undress each other. I continued to hold my pee. Soon, he was just in his boxer shorts and black dress socks and I in nearly nothing. I lay sprawled out on the bed and considered getting up to go to the bathroom. But I couldn't do it! I was too embarrassed! And that's when it happened. Matthew, being completely unaware of my inner turmoil, seductively reached his hand down and slipped it underneath the soft cotton of my underwear. My cunt felt wet and ready. And so did my thighs. And quickly his fingers felt strangely wet as well. It became immediately obvious to both of us that this warmth spreading over us was not your typical vaginal lubrication, but was instead a steady stream of urine, wetting my body and his, plus his expensive Egyptian cotton sheets, and eventually moving all the way down to his $800 queen-sized mattress. I was pissing everywhere. I lay in my self-made yellow pool for half a second and determined that there was no way to recover from this. I stood up, muttered an apology, pulled my jeans on over my damp legs, and fled.

To his credit, Matthew called me for weeks afterward. He would leave reassuring messages on my answering machine, telling me not to worry and asking me to call him back. Less to my credit, I never did. If my approach to learning sex was trial by fire, I considered Matthew a raging blaze that I was not willing to put out. I took from him the reminder to always, always pee (in the toilet), and I walked away with a bit more baggage.

I wish I could say that this was it, that I could rub my palms together, slap my hands on my knees, and say: "Well, that's all, folks. That is the entirety of my fumbles, bumbles and flounders as I have stepped ungracefully into my sexuality. I have laid all my truths out before you." But in actual fact I could go on and on and on, seemingly without end. Sex has never come easily to me. It has not been intuitive, natural, or graceful. It has been hilarious, thought-provoking, and full of hard lessons, but it has never looked the way that I thought it was supposed to.

I have found myself in these situations not because I am not good at this kind of thing, nor is it a result of my disability. My teenage worries were misplaced, and it proved untrue that being disabled would make sex difficult for me. No, I have achieved these mishaps because I was largely misinformed about the nature of sex. Like many of us, I was misled to believe that there was some kind of formula, a trajectory we were all supposed to know and to follow. I naively took the images of sex taught to me by movies, TV, and porn as truth. I believed that I was supposed to move seamlessly from being clothed to being penetrated and that it would always result in simultaneous orgasms and that I would always enjoy it. Without any sort of sex education (notwithstanding Katherine and her melons), nor a space where I could ask difficult and vulnerable questions, I was left to make false assumptions. The silence around sex steers us in dark directions. And so it is only through experiences that I have come to realize that there is in fact no specific procedure, no right way of doing it. I know now that sex can look a million and one different ways. I have luckily discovered that I do not have to fit my disabled body into an able-bodied portrait of erotic intimacy. I can create my own framework and choose my own desires.

I think that for many of us, at many points in our lives, the sex we are having does not match our idea of what it is supposed to be like. Our imaginations are unrealistic, informed as they are by movies and porn and unattainable standards of beauty. I don't think I am alone in finding out that sex can be uncomfortable and clunky. And that is exactly why I do the work that I do. I am involved in sex education because I could have really used some education of my own at various points in my life. I would have been saved years of anxiety and confusion if someone had sat me down and talked to me about our bodily mechanics. My early sex life would have been vastly different if I had other people with disabilities as role models. If I had known that all people sometimes pee and bite and fart when they don't mean to, I would have been spared a lot of sleepless nights. If there weren't so much shame and silence all caught up around sex, then maybe I would have been able to ask someone all of my deep, dark questions. But I wasn't.

So here I am now, truthfully and shamelessly telling you this:
I have mistakenly tried to eat a penis.
I have accidentally peed on an adult man.
I have farted, loudly, right in that beautiful moment
of orgasm.
I have said the wrong thing at absolutely every chance.
I have giggled instead of groaned,
have gagged instead of gushed.
I would prefer to be honest. May all my inexpert errors
reassure you: you are not alone.

FRESH-FACED AND ORGASM FREE

I woke up this morning and got myself off. It is an exercise I have been trying to implement more and more into my daily life. Some people take up meditation, others cut out gluten. But to me increased masturbation seems like the ticket to a less stressful, more happy and healthy life. I am writing this in the grey days of January, when the new year is affording us some hopeful vigour despite the fact that winter is only just getting its footing. The ambition of our collective resolutions is in the air and I am taking it all to heart, or rather to my bits. I have seven sex toys lined up beside my bed along with a bottle of lube. Multi-coloured and pretty, they stand at attention, offering me promises of pleasure. I have been making sure that at least four times a week, I begin my day by reaching out to them. It would be quicker not to. My days are full and it would seem that the most practical way to start them would be with coffee and typing. But getting up for the immediate click-click-click of fingers on keys proves depressing. I do it but I don't like it. And so instead, I treat myself to these four wake-ups with alternative technological objects.

I am not quick. I have never been quick. These morning masturbations are drawn out. I need at least forty-five minutes to reach my climactic end goal, and that is with my vibrators. Those people who can rub one out in the bathroom stall on their lunch break—that has never been me. When I'm fucking myself, it is a lengthy endeavour. I've been practicing for years and still my body remains resistant to my fingers, demanding substantial time and attention before being charmed. I've accepted it. I'm just not easy.

It has always been this way for me. I did not begin my work at a sex shop as an orgasm aficionado. As indicated by my aforementioned cringeworthy exploits, I did not always play well with others. Unfortunately, I was not so skilled at playing with myself either. At the time that I was hired by Venus Envy—the sex shop where I now work—I had experienced roughly two orgasms in my entire life thus far (one from a man named Thor, which is a whole other story, and one by my own hand, after about an hour of some strenuous digital explorations). It sometimes feels like a fluke that I was hired at all. But they gave me a chance and here I am.

I got the job at Venus Envy the summer I turned twenty-three. I had just graduated with a liberal arts degree and I was looking for absolutely any sort of work I could find. I had papered the town with resumes repeatedly and had only gotten two call-backs. Coincidentally they were both for work at high-end, tourist-driven candy shops, neither of which hired me. Apparently I had not had enough "experience with candy." My options were seeming pretty bleak when Venus Envy called me in for an interview. I was terrified.

I had applied at the store with absolutely no expectations. Venus Envy is an award-winning, education-based sex shop, a pillar of Halifax's queer community, and the only place of its kind east of Toronto. Considering it has such credentials, I assumed the staff were required to come armed with a few of their own, none of which I believed I had. I lacked a background in sexual health, I did not identify as queer (yet), and thus far I had not had a single moment of purely enjoyable, uncomplicated sex. It appeared as though the odds were against me. Yet I had applied all the same. It seemed like a dream job and I had to try.

Here I must confess: I was not initially so wildly interested in working at a sex shop because I cared a lot about sex. At this point in my life I had stopped even thinking about it much. My attempts at doing it (both alone and with others) having largely failed me, it would be fair to describe my lusty feelings as being in remission. Sex was not the driving force behind my bold job application. The truth is, I was most interested in the books. Venus Envy has the very best books. The shelves seem endless. Pages and pages of new fiction, feminist publications, and cultural critiques line the walls of the store. I wanted to dive into all of them. I wanted to get lost in Venus Envy's literature, take each shiny new paperback home and make it my own. Working there seemed to be the best way to make this happen. I was in it for the books, not the dildos. And I really wanted in.

I went to the interview dressed in my most professional-looking outfit. I chose clothes that I thought would make me look more sexually seasoned, imagining I would be judged on my personal history. I also preemptively constructed anecdotes that I hoped would make me appear mature, confident, and experienced. I had even gone so far as to study some anatomical diagrams online the night before, in case the interview had a pop-quiz component. I furtively reviewed the names of all the parts, mouthing the words "labia majora," "pubic mound," and "frenulum," in my bedroom while my roommates watched the baseball game on TV just outside the door.

It turned out that all my efforts had been in vain. The interview was easy. I did not have to reference my sexual history nor answer any multiple choice questions. My orientation and prowess, or lack thereof, were irrelevant. I was only required to chat with my soon-to-be-boss, who seemed pretty great. We talked mostly about my retail experience and whether or not I liked doing things like dusting and reshelving stock. It was all pretty straightforward and I felt confident I had come off appearing pretty normal, perhaps even capable and charming. I had. I got the job and started work a week later.

I loved it immediately. It felt perfect for me from the very start. Talking about sex came easily. Someone would walk in and uncomfortably browse the shelves for forty-five minutes before timidly admitting that they wanted to purchase their first sex toy. Or someone would saunter in nonchalantly and tell me that they needed a bigger butt plug. Groups of teen-age boys, old lovers, queer couples, baffled husbands, mothers and daughters—they all came in, feeling anxious or at home or sometimes unaware of what they were walking into. I loved helping all of them.

Working at a sex shop is a job of hearing secrets and holding truths, of trying to alleviate weight from people's shoulders and shame from people's chests. It felt like an honour to be doing it. And despite my own lack of sexual experience and orgasmic difficulties, I was good at it. I was a good listener. And providing advice and information that could mitigate someone's fears or fulfill their desires was simple. I just had to repeat all that I had been taught in my training and mimic the vernacular of my co-workers.

"This toy is made of 100% medical-grade silicone, which is great, because it means it can be sterilized."

"This toy is well-shaped for external stimulation. The clitoris has 8,000 nerve endings, which means that vibrations can feel really awesome, or, of course, not awesome at all, because all bodies are different."

"When buying your first butt plug, you should start small, make sure your toy has a base, and always add a lot of lube."

It was all a matter of repetition and friendly delivery. For the first few months it felt easy. People would ask questions and I would listen attentively and then recite a response. No problem. Until one day it stopped being easy. And then everything felt like a problem.

It was about my sixth month into it. I had been working at the shop for long enough to begin feeling totally comfortable there. The job was as dreamy as I had imagined it would be: I was allowed to borrow whichever books I wanted and even read them in the shop if there were no customers around. I was eating words for breakfast, consuming feminist theory at a rapid pace. I was all alone in the shop and immersed in a queer fiction novel when the customer walked in.

They[2] looked about my age, maybe a few years younger. Blonde hair spilled asymmetrically around their face and an old backpack, held together with patches, was slung across their shoulders. They entered the store and immediately ducked behind a bookshelf without looking up. From where I was standing, I could see that they were chewing the skin around their thumb and closely examining the toe

---

2. I use the pronoun "they" rather than "he" or "she" because I would not want to make assumptions about anyone's gender.

of their left boot rather than the book spines before them. These were all the telltale signs of a nervous customer, and so I allowed them their space.[3]

For half an hour I puttered around them while they lifted boxes of tampons, examined bottles of lube, and put each item back down before stuffing their hands hard into their pockets. I said hello at one point, but they ignored me, or maybe didn't hear me. As they continued their meandering explorations of the shop, they moved closer and closer to the back wall. The back wall is many people's site of anxiety. Dozens of sex toys lean upright in their shelves. Above the vibrators hang tough-looking black leather harnesses. From one corner protrude twenty dildos with names like Outlaw, Tsunami, and Buck. While we try to make the space as welcoming as we can, given the titillating nature of sex toys, it is difficult to mediate some people's reactions. A lot of folks respond to a wall of dildos by immediately grabbing a cock and engaging their friends in a dildo sword fight. Others, like this person, seem not to want to be near it. I am more partial to the timid kind of customer myself. This is the customer I can most relate to, as someone who has also been daunted by sex. So I was not too concerned about being able to help this nervous shopper. I knew I would be able to get them what they wanted.

They finally reached the rear of the shop and stood in front of the vibrating bullets with their arms crossed tightly over their chest. I approached them.

"Do you need help finding anything today?" I asked,

---

3. It should be noted that this customer is a construction. Staying true to the Unofficial Pact of Sex Shop Workers, I would never, ever, disclose information about any person who came into the store. This nervous customer is a made-up version of someone who could be real, and this experience is an exaggerated account of some things that could happen.

trying to sound especially congenial. They shook their head no, without looking at me.

"Okay, cool," I continued with a chipper voice. "Well, these toys all have batteries in them so you can feel them in your hands if that's helpf—"

The customer's confession exploded from their mouth and cut me off. Their words were rushed and jumbled.

"I can't orgasm. I have been trying my whole life and I've just never done it. My friends say they do it all the time and they think I'm a weirdo. They even squirt! I must be like, broken down there or something, right?" They gestured downward.

Their face was pale and they seemed so worried that I immediately empathized. I knew this feeling. And I believed I knew how to reassure this person, having heard my co-workers address concerns like this many times before. I started into a comforting spiel, offering generic pieces of advice and platitudes. I talked about how all bodies are different, how we all need different lengths of time, different pressure, different toys, and different types of stimulation. I was repeating this all by rote and I could tell that it was working.

Comforted, the customer tentatively looked at toys with me. After we selected one we moved on to books, and I pointed out some helpful orgasm guides that my co-workers had told me were the most informative. Lastly, we chose a bottle of lube to accompany the vibrator. As we selected items, I watched the customer's shoulders move away from their ears and saw their face open up. They were visibly letting their guard down and I felt satisfied that I was doing a good job.

It was as we were finishing up, while I swiped the debit card and bagged the items, that the customer asked me the most difficult of questions: "So these things worked for you, right?"

I had never been asked this before. A skill you learn when working in a sex shop is to deflect attention away from yourself. You are only an anonymous sounding board for other people's personal narratives. Therefore, my sexual experiences and preferences had never been dragged into the mix. This was a whole new situation and I was unsure how to proceed.

I am a terrible liar, and the truth was that these things had not worked for me. I had not even tried to make anything work for me. I had been employed at Venus Envy for half a year and I had been spending all of my paycheques on books. My library had certainly evolved, but my capacity to experience pleasure had remained stagnant. I had not even really been thinking about sex at all. It sounds absurd, I know, considering I was talking about it every day. But I was never talking about *my* sex; I was only listening to the sex stories of others. I was learning how to be a good listener, not a good lover. I had perhaps even subconsciously not been reflecting on my own sex life, disappointing as it had been. When you spend all day talking to people who are doing some sort of fucking, it can be depressing to remember that you are not. But now I was being directly asked about it and there was nothing I could do but lie.

"Yeah, uh, definitely. Definitely did. These are, uh, these are some great, uh, great things ya got here. Great stuff." I responded hesitantly, trying to sound vague and appear self-certain.

When the customer left, I sat down, floored by the full-on recognition that I still knew nothing about coming from a personal standpoint. For months now, I had been talking the practicalities of sexual satisfaction, waxing poetic on sex toys as if I knew their value. But all I was doing was regurgitating rather than speaking from any actual experience. On the plus side, I no longer wasted much time worrying about sex. I had stopped actively examining all of my long-standing sex-related neuroses. But this was not because I had worked through them. I had just stopped thinking about them! I had simply stuffed all of my concerns haphazardly under the rug. The bulging bulk of them was suddenly apparent.

Since starting work at Venus Envy, I had not masturbated, had not orgasmed, and had not used the one single vibrator I had ambitiously purchased on my first day of work. The pink, jelly, phallic object had been lying fallow in my underwear drawer for months now. The limitations posed by this experiential absence were suddenly feeling noteworthy. There would be times, I realized, where having actually done something myself would make it much easier to talk about that thing. While I was not about to delve into the depths of bondage and spanky play for the sake of work (yet), I figured I should at least try to learn how to give myself an orgasm. It seemed a suitable preliminary skill to have.

It was not as though I had never tried to fwap one out before. I had thoroughly examined my stuff below the belt and had found it (sort of) fun on (just) one occasion. But for the most part, my explorations of my Southern Hemisphere had found more valleys than peaks. No matter how hard I pressed, how long I rubbed, whether I up-stroked, down-stroked or kept it a little to the left, almost all of my results had been anticlimactic. I was not sure what I was doing wrong, but clearly something was not right.

It could be that I was disabled. Just as I had worried that a spinal cord injury would keep me from knowing how to fuck others, I also worried that it would keep me from feeling good on my own. Since the accident I had been back and forth from doctor to doctor many, many times. At each examination I had been subjected to enough tests with the Wartenberg wheel to know that my sensation was limited. With my eyes closed, the doctors would prick my legs with needles, press hot and cold objects to my toes, and rub the wheel along my skin. Their touches would resonate as ghostly tingles. I knew something was there but I did not know exactly what. The doctors would peer down over their noses at me lying prostrate on the white, papered examination table and label me a "four out of five." They would send me home without explaining what that meant. I knew not to test water temperature with my toes, but I imagined it all must have some larger-scale consequences than an inability to determine the tepidness of pool water with my feet. Perhaps part of the repercussions was that those 8,000 nerve endings in my clit were not operating to their full capacity? Maybe my so-called "magic button" was not so magic after all? Maybe this was why I had never really gotten all hot and bothered from touching it?

Or maybe the problem was simply a lack of imagination. I had learned my vulva through the least sexy framework possible: the medical lens. I sustained my spinal cord injury at the green age of nine. This meant that I quite quickly learned all about my body as though it were a problem, something that I had to learn to work with and rehabilitate. I grew to know my junk as something that would leak urine and that I had to take care of by frequently catheterizing. I learned all about my urethral opening and how to insert a lubricated plastic tube into it long before I knew what the clitoris was or what sorts of things could feel good in other holes. My vulva was simply another part of my disability, and it was a place I knew intimately in that context. Every time I went to the bathroom, I would gently spread open my labia to insert the catheter. Touching myself was so common that it was hard to imagine it as a sexual experience. It was functional, not hot. Necessary, not fun. Maybe it was this long-standing pattern that was holding me back, and to get the goods out of masturbating, I had to work on some reprogramming? Could that be my wrong turn?

Regardless of what the root problem was, the outcome had been that I had, at some point, accepted that I was one of those women who "just couldn't." But my experience with the customer had called this thesis into question. I decided to extend the kind reassurances I issued to others to myself as well. I was ready to revisit my cunt. And predictably, I decided to begin with books.

At work, we have an entire shelf dedicated to the female orgasm. I diligently brought home a copy of every single volume. Beginning with *The Elusive Orgasm* and moving all the way through to *Slow Sex,* I searched the pages. For weeks, the stack sat beside my bed and I plowed through it every night. I dog-eared pages and highlighted pointers. I was an industrious scientist, a dedicated student. I was trying to somehow draw out a map of what I should do to successfully come. I wanted to figure out what approach to best take when butterin' my muffin.

I was looking specifically for experiences like mine, for heartening anecdotes and some validation. I suppose what I needed was something like *Chicken Soup* for the vulva. That is not exactly what I found. Instead, I discovered some really helpful information, but also some questionable constructs. While it was great to read about anatomy and technique, something in these pages was not resonating with me.

In some books, the problem was the oft-repeated sentiment that you would "just know." This indefinite stock phrase was so lacking that it felt more like a misdirection than a guide post. If one is in search of something hard to find, they need some clear markers that they are on the right path, not to be told to just follow their intuition. Telling everyone that they would all "just know" implies that all orgasms feel the same for all people. Orgasms always feel like something so indefinable they can't be described?! I didn't buy it. If it was true that everyone liked different kinds of sex (and my work at the shop had definitely affirmed this truth) then it must also follow that everyone experiences orgasms differently. I resented the amorphous homogeny that so many of these orgasm guides were putting forth.

In other texts, the obvious problem was the focus put on partnered sex and penetration. I had stopped trying to find my sweet spot at someone else's hand long ago. I knew from experience that having somebody or something in me was not a sure way to success, so I immediately disregarded any advice that indicated that I should get my partner to touch me in all the right places and put things in me. My orgasm would not be codependent, thank you.

But there was something more to it than these simple shortcomings. Something else was not fitting quite right; there was some sort of larger structural issue at play. It took me a while but eventually I was able to pinpoint it. The problem was that none of this stuff made room for my disability. Every sex expert, masturbating master and intimacy theorist, whose writing I was reading, was operating under the assumption that I, the reader, was able-bodied.

"Simply move your fingers in rapid, circular motions

around the clitoris," the author would write, presuming that moving one's fingers was always "simple."

"The clitoris will swell and protrude when stimulated." These accounts didn't take into consideration that perhaps not every clitoris was necessarily capable of swelling.

"You should feel your vagina contract," stated one book. But could my vagina contract? What muscles made it contract? Could those muscles be affected by my disability? And what would those contractions feel like?

The assumption of able-bodiedness meant that almost all of the informative orgasm guides I was reading left me with more questions. None of these books were speaking to my experience. It occurred to me that perhaps I had yet to learn my way of coming because all the step-by-step methods I was reading, all the porn I had watched, and all the sex I had had thus far had not considered my disability. Everything I had read, watched, and done had been about being able-bodied, something I was just not and did not want to be.

It reminded me of the way I had been taught to stand up out of a chair. All the doctors and rehabilitation experts would tell me not to use my strong arms to pull myself upright. They would encourage me to practice engaging my core, to use my quads, to rely on my ankles. This was the "correct" way of standing up. But the abilities of my core, quads and ankles have always been dubious. They are not my strongest assets, while my biceps have always been highly over-developed. I had long ago stopped listening to all the specialists. I was very happy using my arms to pull myself up off the couch or the kitchen chair. When they all described to me the "correct" way of doing something, they were using "correct" as synonymous with "able-bodied." But my disabled way of moving worked just fine for me, and

I was not interested in rehabilitating myself so that I could better conform to a normative way of being. I loved my difference. I believed—still believe—that the most beautiful part of residing in difference is that you get to reconstruct everything we are told is truth and build for yourself a way of being that fits for you. The way I stand up with my arms is fabulous, the way I carry things in my teeth rather than my hands is magnificent, and the way I drag my right foot is spectacular. Each of those movements collide and create a way of moving through the world that is the most efficient for me. I had learned to disregard therapists who had tried to correct me and ignore anyone who described a "proper" way of doing something.

I decided to apply this attitude to fucking myself. It was such a relief to realize that just as there is not one right way of getting up and down the stairs, there is not one right way of getting off. I approached my newfound masturbatory practice with this as my mantra. Realizing that none of the paths had been constructed in my favour freed me to bushwhack my own path and follow my own particular swaying and zigzagging way to my destination. My jerk-off practice was a deconstruction site. I was reworking everything.

I went home from work each night and practiced. My self-love sessions were long-winded, to say the least. With absolutely every part and position now becoming a potential pleasure zone, the variables I could try at feeling good were endless. I put toys in all new places. Nothing was off-limits. I worked my way through bottles and bottles of lube and brought home a plethora of new toys. My bedside table was no longer laden with books but with butt plugs (and dildos and nipple clamps and vibrators). I was willing to try everything and anything in the name of figuring myself out.

And the best part about all of this was that my new efforts were not being undertaken out of fear, anxiety or a pressure to be "normal." Instead, my bodily explorations, now un-encumbered from an ill-fitting and able-bodied standard, held the potential for all sorts of magic.

I grew up my desires and the shape of my sex in that way, on my own terms. I did not follow others' advice but developed my own strategy. And it did not happen "just like that." I cannot write that one night my clandestine attempts at coming bore fruit and I was ushered into the secret society of Women Who Come. It would perhaps be easier to write that I eventually put all the right things in all the right spots and there it was, just like that—I "just knew."

But that would be completely untrue. Of course it did not work that way. All my late-night loving taught me a lot, but it didn't teach me to be a sure thing. My cunt still needs to be wooed. I still have to practice four times a week. I cannot just roll over and get myself off in a hot minute before I enter into my day. And then when I do come, I do not know exactly if it feels like it is supposed to feel. I do not know if it feels the way yours feels, or those of the person to your left. I am willing to bet we all orgasm differently, considering we all have different parts. My coming is all my own. My orgasms are unpredictable and hard to define. They are not marked off or delineated. Instead, my body tumbles in and out of feeling good, just as it tumbles in and out of being upright. I trip into coming.

So I woke up this morning and got myself off. Today it took roughly forty-five minutes, and I did it exactly the way I wanted to.

THE LADY & THE BUTCH

I heard the tell-tale ding-dong of our door and looked up. I had been completely absorbed in my book, the store having been empty for the last hour and a half. It was one of those wet, grey days that are so painfully commonplace in Halifax. The damp cold will seep into your bones and make a bomb shelter there, securing itself inside your very core for the duration of the winter. Nobody was going to leave their house and come to a sex shop that afternoon. I was willing to bet that no one was even having sex, anywhere, in the entire city. We were all too depressed as a population, oppressed as we were beneath the low-slung metallic sky. So I gave myself to the pages of books, certain that I had the day to myself.

Two people entered into the warmth of the shop and my surprise deepened. They seemed like an unlikely pair to be coming into a sex shop together. The taller person brought up the rear, squeezing their broad shoulders through the door. I noticed them first, admittedly not because of their height but because they were a stone-cold fox. Their hair, cut short against their scalp, seemed to have partially frozen in the winter's air, some strands turned icy silver amongst the dark crop. They were wearing a work suit, faded brown with a zipper up the front and dirt rubbed deep into the knees. Their hands were big and bare, turned red in the chill and tightly curled around the back handles of a wheelchair. They pushed the chair forward with a confident strut, a swagger often attributed to butches of a certain generation. The other person led the way in their chair. This person was older, I would have guessed somewhere in their eighties or early nineties. Their skin had that translucence associated with the old age we are all approaching, veins appearing as bulging rivers on their skin's pale surface. This person was quite small, seeming delicate and fragile. Most of their body was protectively enclosed in a purple, floral print, one-piece snow suit. Topping all of this was a tightly curled crown of hair which has been dyed a shade of mauve, perfectly complimenting the suit.

Despite the older person's small stature and presumed fragility, I could hear them assuredly barking orders at the person they were with, their voice captured by that particular rasp induced by years of cigarette smoking. "Move me in here faster! I am nearly dead from all this goddamn fucking cold, Janet!" They declared, as the other person, whom I now knew to be Janet, pushed them inside. This monologue of complaints continued as the two slowly approached the counter. Janet, for their part, continued to say nothing.

I put my book down and smiled, prepared to help the pair, but also already feeling a little fearful of this brash and seemingly tough-as-fuck elderly person. I felt certain I could not be subjected to such sternly issued commands and maintain as confident a strut and posture as Janet.

The two reached me, and with eyes level to the counter, the older one glared at me. My saccharine smile was not fooling anyone. This person could smell my hesitation and uncertainty. Their sharp blue eyes could pierce through the standardized store clerk demeanor to my very soul. They looked me up and down.

"Well, tell her, Janet," the purple-clad person ordered.

I turned my eyes up to Janet. This person also seemed to be able to see into my soul and read my mind, which was unfortunate, because at that moment my mind was entirely consumed with some pretty dirty thoughts about them. Janet cocked their eyebrow, smirked, and reached into the front pocket of the faded work suit. They pulled out a credit card and threw it down on the counter.

"Get this woman whatever she wants. Price don't matter."

The directions were clear and authoritative and Janet's voice was clipped, as though they would prefer not to speak at all, but instead to enforce order with a look and a shrug of their shoulders. I briefly wondered how these two seemingly domineering people could ever get along.

I nodded obediently and then turned my gaze to the older woman. She stared at me with menace in her eyes, daring me to try and talk to her about sex.

I shifted my focus again, intending to issue a pleading stare toward Janet, but they were already sauntering to the door, their broad back to me. Appearing to sense my look of doubt, Janet turned and came back to us.

"My number," they said, laying a post-it on the counter with seven digits scrawled messily across it. Shit! Janet *had* read my fucking mind and now they were coming on to me in front of their grandmother?! I blushed and then gave a knowing smirk of my own.

"To call me. When she's through. So I can pick her up," Janet explained. I blushed redder, swallowed the smirk off my now-sheepish face, and nodded.

Janet left, squeezing through the door. I turned to the older woman. Her arms were folded across her small chest, and she looked a little like a withered concord grape, sour through and through. I almost laughed.

"She's my granddaughter-in-law. She's one of those lesbians," she rasped. I nodded. I had been exclusively bobbing my head since this duo had come in, feeling unsure of my ability to form any sort of coherent sentence. My neck was feeling tired.

"Are you a queer? You sure don't look like much of one," she asked. I mean, I suppose she was asking a question, but it felt more like she was giving me some kind of back-handed compliment, one of the homophobic variety. Either way, she was right. I sure don't look like much of a queer. My hair is entirely symmetrical, falling in blonde curls halfway down my back. I have no face piercings. No telling ring hangs from my septum. My tattoos are easy to hide and my clothes are feminine. Sometimes this may mean I fall victim to femme invisibility, but it also means that I can pass. I can pass as straight, dodging homophobia with my gender-conforming, heteronormative presentation. And this was a moment where I considered doing just that. I so badly wanted to avoid the ridicule of this terrifying granny that I almost, for a split second, thought about lying. But lying would be a gross act of cowardice, reinforcing what I perceived to be bigotry. I could not do that. So instead I nodded. Again.

"Hmmm," she grunted. And then she surprised me by saying, "good. I prefer that. My granddaughter is a queer lesbian and she knows all about sex. Lesbians always do, you see. It is their specialty," she continued, "or so I am told. Me, I'm definitely not one of 'em. I was married to the same man for forty-six years. My Darrel. He died twenty-three years ago and I haven't let no hand touch me since. Not even my own. Thought it would be unfaithful."

At this point her eyes welled up. I could see a crack in her purpled, hardened front. I went to reach my hand out to hers, covered in age spots and clasped on the countertop, but before I could interject with a touch or some sort of re-assurance, she pulled her hands back and continued.

For twenty minutes, she told me all about Darrel, his work as a mechanic, his love of dogs, her love of him, and the babies they raised together. It was one long, linear narrative, full of the most caring details and all delivered in her contrary bark of a voice. It was as if prefacing her purchase with the story of her loved one would soothe her guilt, would cancel out the infidelity she believed she may be perpetrating. Eventually she concluded with her reason for being here in front of me.

"So now Susanne, my granddaughter, Ronny's eldest, and Janet there, her wife, say I need to buy a dildo. They know all about them, you see, because they are queer lesbians. They say if I just have some fun and let loose a little for a minute I won't be so cranky all the time. Sus even thinks it'll help with my arthritis, but to that I say she's one of those woo-woo hippie weirdos who don't know a goddamn thing. Anyway, here I am, I suppose, and you better fix me up." It was an order, and one I was sure I could fill.

There are moments, such as when this older woman and her granddaughter-in-law had walked in, when I feel intimi-dated. It is nerve-wracking to have strangers walk up to you and unload their sexual baggage, asking you for answers, for the cure-all vibrator, for a way to feel good. I wonder, for a second, who am I to have these solutions? I am young! I am relatively inexperienced! I know nothing! But then I remember that no one really expects me to have the right answer. There often isn't one at all.

All people need is an ear. They just want to talk. These conversations are not happening anywhere else. It is so difficult to have a sexual question or concern and not have someone to talk to about it. I calm down, remember my role, and I listen.

The woman and I walked over to the wall of sex toys, all of them charged and lined up for her to inspect. We perused vibrators, dildos, nipple clamps, and cock rings. She held the vibrators in her hands, laughing a hoarse yap as they buzzed against her fingertips. She asked me the standard questions: Which one is the best one? Which one do you like? Do women really buy these things? I answered each to the best of my ability and eventually she settled on a cute battery-powered vibe in her favourite colour (purple).

Back at the counter, I rang her through. I put batteries in her toy and made sure it all worked so that when she got home, it would be ready to go. I gave her an information sheet, telling her all about cleaning it. I reassured her that her purchase was entirely normal and very classy and she just might like it. Then I called Janet to let her know we were all finished up.

As we waited for her ride, I tried to make small talk with the older woman, but she was strangely quiet, looking down rather than glaring at me with those penetrating blue eyes. I thought perhaps she was embarrassed, having just revealed to me some of her more intimate secrets. But then she said, "let me see that."

I realized she had not been looking down bashfully, but had been intently examining the pride jewellery displayed in the front of our counter. I lifted the glass top and she reached in, pulling a beaded rainbow necklace in between her crooked fingers.

"This is for the gays, right?" She asked me.

"Yeah, the rainbow is a symbol of gay pride."

"I'll take one of these then," she said.

I pulled the rainbow choker out of the case and clasped it around her neck. Janet walked in just as I was holding up a mirror, showing the grandmother how perfectly suited the beads were to her snow suit.

The two smiled at each other. Then the grandmother immediately began the nagging, laying down her laws. "What took you so long, Janet?! I'm nearly dead from how goddamn hot it is in here! Leaving me all alone with a bunch of queer lesbians! You would!"

Janet smiled and almost chortled, obviously impervious to the grandmother's near constant string of complaints and reprimands. They left together, moving as a single unit back out into the cold.

The next week we got a phone call down at the shop. It was my day off, so my co-worker took it. She said an older woman with a raspy voice had called looking for the blonde queer lesbian. She wanted to tell me thank you, and that it was a good choice even though her arthritis is still aching.

I am sure Darrel didn't mind.[4]

---

4. An endnote: Much like the customer who could not orgasm, neither of The Lady nor The Butch are real. They are extrapolations, amalgamations, versions of myself and people I know all blurred together. To reiterate: I would never, ever write about another person's true desires or experiences in the store.

HOW I LEARNED TO STOP WORRYING AND LOVE MY TRICYCLE

Halifax is a city with hills. On bike rides I careen down them, helmet off, trying to attain lightning speeds. Or I crawl up them, slow but sure, breathing heavy. I live on the steepest hill of them all, right at the bottom. This makes my bike ride home the most satisfying part: on the last leg of my journey I don't pedal at all, but hold my legs out as I am propelled down, down, down to my front door, the world a blur of coloured clapboard at my sides and shining ocean ahead of me. Going up on my way to work is more difficult. I push my bike unevenly up, up, up, using my whole body to move its awkward weight.

My bike is heavy. This is because it is really more of a tricycle, a big red bike with "training wheels" attached on the back. I use quotations because they look like training wheels, but they are not. I am not training for anything. They will never be removed and my bike will never be a two-wheeled beast. They will forever be there supporting me, letting me be balanced as I move through the city. I am not, and will never be, stable enough to move on a bike of two wheels. The idea of even sitting on one, with feet placed on pedals so far off the ground, makes me nervous. My weight would shift hopelessly and uncontrollably back and forth and I would be flat on the pavement in one fell swoop.

My body is just not balanced. Instead, it is one beautiful and chaotic mess. Above the waist, I can manipulate my shoulders, arms, hands and fingers with ease. I can turn my neck from left to right and cock my head at will. I can whisper sweet-nothings or scream loud-somethings from my mouth at absolutely any time I want to. This top half of my body is at my mind's command. It is below the waist that things get a little more complicated. The messages moving through my spinal cord to my lower body get jumbled up and mis-shapen on their journey south, making my movements come out jolted. The idea of walking that I hold in my head is lost in translation and my legs, being unable to interpret my mind's intentions, scissor in and out. My hips sway back and forth and my toes drag slowly against the ground. It is not balanced. What comes out is a way of moving my body that is subject to trips and falls and unpredictable veers. But what I lack in balance I make up for in grace. Trust me: these differences are not to be pitied nor looked down on, and definitely not "righted." They are completely right, in all of their disarray. They disallow me from riding a two-wheeled bike, maybe, but the bike I have now is more perfect than anything I could have imagined anyway.

This bike was built for me by a boy named Bobby, whom I thought I was in love with for one hot minute one hot summer. We spent the late nights of August kissing in parks, on stoops, and in our bedrooms. In the mornings I would leave his house, lips raw, and he would watch me bike away, very slowly, on a bike inherited from my grandfather. The bike I rode back then was one built for the elderly, to be maneuvered through the flat lanes of Florida's trailer park retirement communities. The seat was huge, made for a butt at least five times wider than mine. That big seat was surrounded by three equally big wheels, one out front and two in the back. It weighed a tonne, took corners at dangerously teetering angles, and forced me to move at a crawl no matter how hard I pedaled.

Bobby was a bike mechanic, and he took it upon himself to build me something better. It took him a few months to complete his project, and he surprised me with the new bike right before the winter set in. It was an incredible surprise. Bright red and lightweight, I fell in love with it immediately. The small wheels he had attached on the back of a regular, two-wheeled road bike were light but still strong enough to keep me balanced. Affixed to the bike by springs, they cornered smoothly and sturdily. I could now move much faster up and down hills, around bends and over speed bumps. I felt powerful, freed, and newly mobile in a way that only those who have had their mobility compromised can truly understand. To be able to cross distances and get to places that I could never have reached before—it was a fucking dream.

If I am going to be honest, I do remember that there was one small moment of uncertainty. Upon receiving the gift, I had a fleeting feeling of doubt, a passing sense of shame that rose up from those dark recesses of myself. Bobby looked at me, proud of what he had built, hoping that I would love it and I did wonder, "what will people think?" For a minute I worried about how people would react when they saw a grown woman careening through city streets with training wheels. But then I swallowed that shame down and left it to rot in my guts. Fuck it. Everyone can kiss my ass, I decided. I have *always* looked different. I will *always* be different. This will never change, and even though there are times when it is difficult, I have made it my own personal project to never be ashamed of myself. To love all of my differences boldly. To never hide nor be silent. I do not want to be quietly disabled, trying to fit in and absorb myself into an able-body-centric world. Just as I do not want to be quietly sexual, pretending I do not do that thing that so many of us do (or at least think about doing). I fuck, and I love, and I move through this world as a woman with a disability. And I will do it all while riding a bright red tricycle. I decided all of this in thirty seconds while Bobby watched my reaction. I made my choice, kissed him, and said truthfully that I loved it. I threw my legs over that bike and rode it all across town.

It's four years later and I'm still hopelessly in love with my bike, if not Bobby. I am still pushing it up hills and propelling it down them, biking to and from work, going back and forth from dinner parties to dance parties. But it is not always easy. My training wheels may keep me balanced and shield my skin from the cuts and scrapes of unforgiving pavement, but they cannot protect me from people's commentary. And while sticks and stones can break my bones, words can break my heart.

It was a sunny Sunday morning and I was biking to a breakfast date. I had spent the earlier hours of that morning in bed with my girlfriend. I had just moments ago let her hands love every inch of my skin, and so as I biked, I felt nothing but worshipped. Sure that everyone would see that I was glowing, I pedaled uphill confidently. The hill was slight, but I was still moving slowly and working hard, my body shifting from side to side. The street was closed to traffic due to a marathon running through the centre of town and the empty expanse felt free and open, just for me. I was just getting into a flow, pedal rotating smoothly after pedal, when I heard the snickers. Three men were to my right, drinking beers on their stoop in the morning sunshine. I turned to them as I heard one say, "isn't it time to take off your training wheels?" I almost stopped. I was not hurt, just annoyed. I felt almost compelled to explain to him why my "training wheels" are important and why I will never take them off. But as the men stared blankly back at me, I decided they were not worth the time. I was hungry, and late for breakfast. I didn't really give a fuck what they thought either way. I kept biking, but as I moved away, I heard them laughing at my back. I heard one say, "look at the way she's moving,"and I thought I heard another use the word "retard." As I peeked back over my shoulder, I saw them mimic my body, as if my unbalances were points of weakness rather than the points of beauty that I perceive them to be.

Comments about my bike are unfortunately not rare. It has turned out that those pangs of worry that I had briefly entertained years ago were entirely accurate. People *do* think that seeing a grown woman with training wheels is a sight to be mocked. The general public *does* seem to believe that my brazen display of difference leaves me open to their criticisms. It is as though I'm asking for it; as if by appearing so proud, I am really just looking to be torn down. Shouts and mutters like those that the men had just issued have happened to me so often that I have developed a certain sort of protection against them. I've got a thick skin and a short-term memory. For the most part, my hide is calloused in all the right places and shields the softer parts of me from ableist comments such as those ones. I most often let slurs slide off my back and arrive at my destination having forgotten them.

But as I biked away from the mocking men, I realized that my thick skin was failing me this time. I felt salt water drip from my tear ducts and into my mouth. My fists were clenched, knuckles white around the handle bars, and my knees wobbled with each rotation. My armour had been punctured and I had no idea what to do about it. I continued heading away from the men, toward the diner. As they became more blurred in the distance, it became clearer and clearer to me that this time, I did not want to shrug it off.

Being impenetrable and impossible to hurt—it doesn't work every time. In fact, always letting ableism slide off my back is dangerous in that it allows ableism to keep happening. I do not want to live in a world where people with disabilities continue to be institutionalized, assaulted, mocked, harassed, and hurt. And when I ignore all the cruel slurs that people hurl at me, then I am, in my acquiescence, permitting this to persist.

I am a disabled person with a whole lot of privilege. I am highly mobile, able to stand upright and ambulate; I am verbal; I do not experience cognitive disabilities. And as I biked away, it fully occurred to me that it was my responsibility to recognize and use this privilege. I did not want to continue to identify as part of a community if I was not going to fight for the rights of that community at all times. I was furious, not because I am not "a retard," but because people who have been labelled "retarded" are a part of my disability community.

I turned my wheel and started to head back toward them, ready to unleash the full length of my anger upon them. I wanted to slap them across the face with my words, make them feel fear with the strength of my vocabulary (those trusted tools of nerds like me, in lieu of fists). But then I thought against it and turned back. This happened three times. I would turn my wheel and then turn it back again. A part of me wanted to scream and kick and rip out hearts and hair. But the more rational part of me was aware that I am small and they were big, I am a disabled woman and they were three able-bodied men, I was shaking with rage and fear and they were probably drunk and self-assured. I knew that no matter the level of my anger, it would be unsafe to go back alone.

So I kept biking and reached the diner. Each turn of the wheel fueled my fury, and by the time I was at breakfast, I was livid. The friends I was meeting had already ordered, and as I walked through the door, fried eggs and buttered toast were being delivered to the table. I slid into the booth at the same moment the plates were plunked down, and immediately tears and snot poured out from my face and onto their morning meals. The breakfast grew cold as I shouted and cried and spewed out all my feelings. As I shared my experience with my friends, my anger snowballed until we were all absorbed in it. We were not to be soothed nor placated. We would pool our collective rage and do something about this.

These friends of mine were three women. As such, none of them were strangers to being yelled at on the street. While I am almost always yelled at for my training wheels, my friends are almost always yelled at for their bodies. When summer starts and soft skin is freshly exposed to warm sunlight, each of us is freshly exposed to patriarchal bullshit. These women, like so many women, cannot leave the house without getting shouted at from cars, cannot go out dancing without feeling that familiar groping of unfamiliar hands on their waists. Their outfits are changed, their routes are reworked, and their movements are limited to avoid those shaming and infuriating catcalls. We have all been subjected to verbal harassment on account of ableism, sexism, and misogyny.

So it was easy to get riled up together. All it took was the drop of one solitary tear and our collective experiences were on the table. We decided to harness those humiliations. This time we would do it all differently. We would not silently be subjected to the hurtful words of others. We would call back. We left our eggs and some crumpled bills and headed back to the stoop where the men had been sitting. We did not have a plan. None of us had ever been in a confrontation like this before. Most often when we are catcalled, we are alone. Most often, the person issuing the shouts is speeding by in a car. This chance to yell back was so rare and we were not sure how to use it. Would the men still be on the stoop? If they were, what would we say? Would we verbally threaten them? Would we stroll on by and catcall them?

We reached the spot to find it empty. This is the part where I would have left. The stoop, littered with beer cans and cigarette butts, intimidated me as it was. I could not imagine how I would feel if the men were still on it. I could not imagine knocking on their door and ushering them downstairs. But before I could turn away, my friend Layla was banging, her fist ringing hard against the wood. One of the people came downstairs. His eyes were bloodshot and his T-shirt stained with grease. He looked disgruntled and stoned.

"What do you want?" he asked us.

"I want to talk to you about the way that you verbally assaulted me earlier," I said politely. Having not prepared well enough, this was what came out. I reverted to being myself:

well-mannered and a little meek. As we had walked over, I had tried to pull up insults from the back of my memory. Half-recalled sentences about beheading and puking down throats had come to mind. They felt too absurd to actually utter. To imagine me, 5'4" and skinny, physically threatening three large adult men was hilarious. It would have been unbelievable and silly, empty threats going nowhere. And so instead I simply asked to speak.

The guy said he did not know what I was talking about. Apparently, he had been outside all morning and no one had "verbally assaulted" anyone. We argued back and forth, him calling me a liar and my friend Layla issuing the obvious statement that no one would make all of this up. Our voices got louder and louder as the asinine debate continued, until eventually his friend, another dude from earlier, came downstairs. He joined the back-and-forth, siding with his buddy that no one had shouted at anyone all day. We all yelled about it until the two men, stating that we were "ruining their brunch," slammed the door.

We did not leave. Instead, we got angrier.

"Fucking cowards!"

"Come down here and face us!"

"Misogynist pigs!" We screamed up to the second floor as we banged and kicked on the door. We were making a scene but we didn't care. All surroundings were forgotten, all social norms thrown out the window. We were a mass of clenched fists, a loud and baleful chorus, a single seething unit. We kept it up as on-lookers uncomfortably hurried by. Eventually, we won out. The two men came back downstairs.

"Look, it was us, okay? I yelled at you about your training wheels. I was stoned and I thought it was funny and I didn't think you would care. Now get over it, okay?" The one with the stained T-shirt issued this begrudged statement of apology as the other one stood silently by him.

I considered this. You might think it absurd that someone could yell at a stranger and then assume that said stranger wouldn't really mind. But actually, I think this seemingly nonsense idea is fully in line with the twisted logic of the patriarchal world we live in. It all makes sense. Within the highly gendered and oppressive culture of North America, women are taught that it is standard for us to be valued based on our physical appearance. If we successfully embody the ideal female archetype, then we will be sexy and desired by the opposite sex. In this imbalanced performance, it is then men's role to aggressively show us that we are successfully desirable by yelling at us, hitting on us, groping us, or eyeing us. Our bodies exist for the viewing. And so catcalling has become so commonplace that we are all supposed to be used to it by now. We should just quit our complaining and consider it a compliment! And while these men were certainly not hurling comments about my sexiness at me, I guess they assumed that I would just be used to being yelled and so I "wouldn't really care."

But that logic doesn't work for me. To me, it does not follow that because I am a disabled woman, I have to accept unsolicited, hurtful commentary from others. When people yell at me as I try to quietly go about my day, it makes me feel unsafe. It reminds me that my fragile skin and small bones can be hurt and broken. It reminds me that my bodily autonomy can be stolen from me at someone else's will. So when the guy stood there and issued his lacklustre apology, I did not forgive him. Instead I stood there, propped up on my four-wheeled bike, and I lectured him.

"I understand that you thought that making fun of me was

funny, but do you understand what it feels like to be yelled at by a stranger on the street? Have you ever been verbally assaulted by someone? Can you imagine what it is like to be a small, disabled woman and to be shouted at by three big men? Would you have yelled at me if I weren't a woman? What if I was bigger than you are and tougher looking? What if I were a man?" Words came out like a flood from my mouth, pooling at our feet right there on Main Street. I was arguing on behalf of myself and all of us who are kettled in by catcalls. It felt like I could go on and on for days and days. The two men, however, were not so absorbed. They silently stood there for a few minutes, but quickly their patience wore thin. They were clearly not being deeply affected by what I perceived to be an extremely eloquent lecture.

"I told you I am sorry, now go home. I don't know what more you want from me," the bigger one said, before he turned away and walked inside. The other one looked at me sheepishly, shrugged and mumbled an apology, and then joined his buddy. They closed the door in our faces.

I turned to my friends, completely unsure of whether I should laugh or cry, feel victorious or defeated. I had been so bowled over by adrenaline that I barely even understood what had just happened, let alone how to respond to it. We went back to the diner and ate breakfast, growing more giddy as we recalled our bravery. But it was not until weeks later that I came to understand that moment as instrumental in helping me access my voice and understand disability.

"Disabled" is such a broad identifier, and having a disability can look so many different ways. If you see me sitting or in photographs you would not necessarily know it. Until you see me walk, you would probably not guess it. All of this means that I pass. I am sometimes assumed to be non-disabled. Riding my trike makes me more visibly disabled. When I am on my trike, I get the most commentary. When I am on "training wheels," people take full liberty to yell at me, tease me, and ask me what's wrong with me. When I let those comments go, left unnoticed, I am allowing them to proliferate. People with different disabilities than mine may experience this kind of verbal harassment more regularly than I do. And so because of my relative position of privilege, I want to make sure I am always using my voice. Having a voice is a right that so many of us are systemically denied access to. I want to make sure I use mine when I can.

The experience of that afternoon did not lead to some kind of seismic shift in the way people see me and my beautiful, red wheels. I still hear the taunts on my rides around town. I rarely respond—not because I don't want to, but more often because it is unsafe. Often the catcaller is driving by and they are gone before I have registered what's happening, or, I am alone and the streets are empty and shouting back seems dangerous. But I will do it again. I am just percolating on my future responses over here, waiting for the perfect moment.

WHAT'S IN A NAME?
MY BIG, WIDE CUNT

I spend a lot of time thinking about words. They are pretty important—we use them to say who we are, what we need, where we are going. They can make or break us. "I am pregnant." "I don't love you." "We are out of toilet paper." These words strung together can really shake up your day.

When it comes to sex in particular, there are lots of words to choose from. We can name our parts cookie, peepee, snatch, schlong, meat stick, or purple-headed monster. We may say we are horny, randy, or turned on. We can assert that we knocked boots, got intimate, or did the nasty. Considering that talking about sex is my job, I think about these kinds of words all the time. I weigh them, massage them with my tongue. The conclusion that these oral examinations have led me to is that a lot of sex-related words don't work for me. They don't match my desires, hug my curves, or fit between my legs. They do not accurately describe the things I do in my bedroom or the part of me that resides between my thighs. This has meant that over the last few years of selling sex toys and writing about sex, my vernacular has inevitably had to shift to better suit my needs. I have reappropriated and refurbished all sorts of words. I have put them in different places and ascribed to them different meanings to make them feel right. By now, I've got my own personal dictionary.

VAGINA VS. CUNT

The dictionary began with the word vagina. Vagina, vagina, vagina. You may think it is an innocuous noun, safely medicalized, and not too risqué. But in my experience, it is a word mired in confusion. Many people don't even know what it means. I myself had been misled about the exact location and identity of the vagina until I was introduced to feminism in my early days of university.

As a sweet, unpoliticized small-town girl, I had been an indifferent vagina-owner for years. I knew what it did and where to find it. It had never caused me much trouble and I felt just fine about it, for the most part. And then one night, early on in my tentative explorations of feminist theory, while flipping through a borrowed, much-used copy of Inga Muscio's *Cunt*, my mind was blown. It was one of those earth-shattering, reality-bending, "Oh, this is why feminism matters!" moments. It was maybe even the catalytic moment that propelled me into becoming the lovely feminist killjoy that I am today. But what is it that I learned, you ask? What is it that forced me to move my hands downwards to protectively cup my junk, that junk I thought I knew, but that I never really knew at all? I learned that the vagina, that *my* vagina, is just a hole! That is all that it defines.

The word "vagina" simply refers to that hole in between your thighs. The fatty lips surrounding the hole: turns out they are not part of the vagina. The nice-feeling nub above the vagina: it has a name of its own. The mound covered in hair: also not a vagina. I had had no idea that all of the sections that make up my junk were not just one entity but were instead a slew of individual, pleasant parts. There were outer and inner labia (those fatty lips) that protected the package. There was a cervix, a weird doughnut-looking thing that hangs out at the back of the vaginal canal. There was a clitoris which seemingly had no function at all, other than to feel really good. And below and in between all of those parts was the vagina, just that little hole. Sure, it's an important hole—one that can push out blood and babies, and can take things in too. But all the same, it remains just one small part of a bigger and more beautiful thing.

Realizing that I had been misinformed about the nature of my body for my entire life thus far really shook me up. I was pissed. It would be just like the patriarchy to limit female bodies like this, I thought. Reducing the sum of our parts to one part totally traps us. A lone focus on the vagina turns us into bodies to be penetrated and bodies that reproduce, and nothing more. It does not recognize our sexual pleasure nor pay homage to our complexities. At the end of the day, calling the sum of our parts our "vagina" hides the reality of the female body's capacity for sexual pleasure.

It follows that the discovery of the true meaning of the word "vagina" next led me to discover "vulva." Vulva. Such a nice, inclusive term. The word vulva refers to the whole damn thing, all of the external genitalia: the clitoris, the inner and outer labia, the vestibule, the mons, the urethra, the vagina. All of it! Vulva is a great word. It is reminiscent of a reliable German car, to be fair, but at least it rolls pretty smooth off the tongue. As a young, wide-eyed, baby wanna-be riot grrrl I fell in love with the word vulva.

If you yourself have ever been an indignant young feminist, or an indignant young anything, endowed with knowledge that is new to you and that you believe to be pivotal and world-changing, then you know how righteous youthfulness can be. I became a vulva zealot. I resolved to use the word vulva as often as possible. I believed that I alone could spread the word to the masses thereby grossly further women's rights. No more shameful euphemisms! No more blanket "vagina"! The vulva would be recognized! No, it would be honoured!

This crusade of mine lasted roughly three months. It took me about that long to realize that shoving the world vulva in people's faces was not dismantling the word order but was only making me look like a big weirdo. This truth became very apparent the day that I chose to tell my sweet, conservative bike mechanic that my bike seat was really hurting my vulva. I stood in front of him with my hands on my hips, wearing the shortest of short-shorts, and made my declaration.

"This bike seat is really making my vulva ache, man."

"Your what?!" he asked.

"My vulva," I repeated.

"I don't know what that is."

"You know, my vagina," I elaborated with a gesture south, even though my vagina was really not part of the problem.

"You mean your front pelvis bone," was his definitive and curt response, issued with a red face and awkward fumbles.

Evidently, a fifty-year-old man does not want to talk to me about my vagina nor learn the anatomically correct name for those parts. Which is understandable, really. So, I decided to drop it. I would call it my vulva should the opportunity arise, but there was no need to bang it over everybody's heads.

Since then, I've stopped using the word vulva. It may be

inclusive of all of my anatomical parts, but it just doesn't work for me anymore. The truth is, it isn't sexy. There is nothing even remotely hot about it. I do not want to tell my lover to touch my vulva, or worse, put her mouth on my vulva. "Baby, put your mouth on my vulva," sounds ridiculous, like I am asking her to taste a jello dish, the kind that has the chunks of stale cake and fruit floating in it. Instead, I've begun using the word cunt. My Big, Wide Cunt is actually what I call it (BWC for short).

Referring to my cunt as big and wide is a coping mechanism my co-worker Holly and I developed. That is what she calls hers too—her big, wide cunt (though I can't say for sure if she acronymed hers as well). We love talking about them, competing over the feats they can accomplish (no matter how exaggerated our claims).

"Dude, last night I had sex with the Vixen Outlaw."[5]

"Whatever, girl, last night my girlfriend fisted me six times and I barely even felt it."

"Yeah, I've done that before. I've also pushed two babies out of my big, fat cunt, so you got nothing."

She always wins the competition. Babies trump everything. But we repeat the same old boasts to each other anyway. I would argue that we *have* to perform this ritualistic pissing contest if only to make sure we're still holding up okay. We have to celebrate the capacities of our cunts, revel in their expansive caverns and love them for their size. We have to argue over whose is bigger and tell each other facetious tales about the things they can hold. If we didn't do this, we may very well be convinced that the opposite is true: that size is bad, that we should want our vaginas to be small and tight.

There is so much messaging in the world telling us that

---

5. The biggest dildo we carry.

there is only one desirable way to be, and we are exposed to this messaging in such a visceral way through our work at the sex shop. You can't talk to people about the most intimate parts of their bodies without being privy to a whole lot of body-shaming attitudes. And we talk to *so many* people who are ashamed of their vulva. They are ashamed of how it looks. They worry that their clit is too big or too small, their labia too droopy or too lopsided, or their pubic hair too dark or too plentiful. They are ashamed of how it smells. Or they are ashamed of what it does and does not do: it does not come fast enough, it excretes too much, it doesn't ejaculate enough. And almost always people are worried that their vaginas are too loose. Being too loose is an ultimate vagina faux-pas in the pornified world we live in.

This shame is not any individual's fault. It makes total sense that women would hate their bodies in a world where we are taught to hate our bodies. Vulvas are to be shaved, douched and tightened, not loved nor left ungroomed. To counter this vehement vulva-policing culture takes a lot of work and repetition. Holly and I have to remind ourselves on the daily that the constructed ideal of femininity is bunk and we don't want that bullshit reaching into the folds of our underwear. We'll keep our cunts as big, wide, and hairy as we please.

FUCKING

Using the word cunt and adding the adjectives "big" and "wide" to the front of it was only the first step in the compilation of my own personalized dictionary. The next step was "fucking." I love the word fucking. Fah-king. The soft start and the harsh, guttural ending make it a perfect word, both as an adjective and a verb. As the former it can be wrathful: "You fucking asshole." Or commonplace: "So I'm talkin' to fackin' buddy over here..." As the latter it can be romantic: "We were fucking and suddenly she paused and told me she loved me." Or insignificant: "Oh yeah, I fucked that guy. It was great." See, it's perfect, able to adapt to all moods and fit all situations. It is the meaning of the verb "to fuck" that I have had to reconsider.

I began thinking about what "fucking" really refers to shortly after starting work at the sex shop. You can't spend your days encountering so many variant human desires and ways of experiencing erotic pleasure and not re-examine your own preconceived notions of what "sex" is. So, in my confusion, I sought Google.

If you turn to the internet, you will find this in the Urban Dictionary:

"In its most literal meaning, fucking refers to the act of sexual intercourse. By extension, it may be used to negatively categorize anything that may be dismissed, disdained, defiled or destroyed."

Yikes! As if dismissed and disdained are "extensions" of sexual intercourse.

To expand on this, let me quote the Wikipedia definition for sexual intercourse: "Sexual intercourse...is chiefly the insertion and thrusting of a male's penis, usually when erect, into a female's vagina for the purposes of sexual pleasure or reproduction; also known as vaginal intercourse or vaginal sex. Other forms of penetrative sexual intercourse include penetration of the anus by the penis (anal sex), penetration of the mouth by the penis or oral penetration of the vulva or vagina (oral sex), sexual penetration by the fingers (fingering), and penetration by use of a strap-on dildo."

Huh. While I sort of appreciate the shout out to queer folks, this definition still leaves me with so many questions. For instance: what if a penis enters my vagina but I don't experience sexual pleasure? What if the penis was only in my vagina for, like, a second? Is there a time limit on this kind of thing? Or what if someone gets off solely through external stimulation and there is no penetration involved? Is it still intercourse if nothing is put in any hole whatsoever? And what if there are four people involved rather than a pairing? Or only one person involved? Is this all a numbers game? Our societal definitions of "fucking" are so limiting. Why does it always have to be about a pair and about penetration? Why does it have to be about genitals at all? By having such a narrow definition, we are only putting restrictions on our ideas about pleasure. We are regulating who has the right to feel good and how.

And so I have redefined the word fucking for myself. I have made it bigger and broader and better. When I write about and think about and talk about fucking, what I am writing about is not penises and vaginas, or penetration, or even orgasms. Fucking, I believe, is an act, and I mean any act, which can be performed alone or consensually with one or more partners, with the ultimate aim of giving and receiving erotic pleasure.

Fucking can mean being stretched out naked on the bed with someone else's hand in your big, wide cunt.

Fucking can mean rubbing your nose against someone else's thigh.

Fucking can mean giving blow jobs.

Fucking can mean masturbating.

Fucking can mean making out.

Fucking can mean breathing deep and thinking the dirtiest of dirty thoughts, if that's how you get off.

The point is that fucking should be about *feeling erotic pleasure*. It should not be about the pressure to orgasm, to make someone else orgasm, to have a partner, or to look hot. If fucking is defined as feeling erotic pleasure, then it can better include all kinds of people, with all kinds of sexualities, bodies, and abilities. I know this is broad, but what's wrong with broad? Why can't we flip our definitions and expand our ideas? It can really only benefit all of us.

This constructed dictionary of mine is not exactly clean. Generally, I feel fine about this. As written at the outset, I am presuming you are not polite company. However, recently I received the following email from my grandmother:

> Hi my dear granddaughter,
>
> I'm sure that I already wrote to comment on your great ability with words in the booklet you wrote. Just saw your Facebook article via Julie's post, and you write really well. You are going to do a superlative job of your book, whatever the topic. My only quibble would be with some language, principally the "F" word because of its shock value. When used in a wonderful part of life that you wish to normalize and make accessible for all, its use may turn away individuals who you are actually anxious to reach. Just a thought from your old Grandmother, who is admittedly, many generations removed from the mainstream in 2013.
>
> –Grandma, 2013

Let me describe to you my grandmother. She is a genius of an eighty-three-year-old woman who can navigate the world of Facebook, blogs and the internet at large. Like grandmothers in fairy tales, she is soft and good for hugging, has filled me with baked goods my entire life, and is endlessly kind. She has never had a drink. She does not smoke nor gamble, nor has she ever had her ears pierced. Having been an elementary school teacher her entire life, she is well-versed in offering supportive and gentle criticisms. In short, I descend from good stock. And imagining her reading my blog makes me cringe with embarrassment.

I considered my grandma's suggestion and realized that she makes a valid point. These words I use do not work for her, or for most people of her generation, many of whom I am sure are having sex and could probably use some sex education (no one knows everything about sex, no matter how old they get). To be fair, if I were speaking with an eighty-three-year-old woman about sex, I would probably not say the word "fucking" to her, nor describe myself as having a big, wide cunt. When writing about sex on the internet, I often imagine my audience as being significantly younger and perhaps more acquainted with my particular style of speech. But my grandmother kindly reminded me that all words have their place, even those that do not match my wants.

When I am sitting at the tiny round table in my kitchen, being vulgar fits best. It makes me feel powerful and tough-as-fuck to control my language. But when I am working in a sex shop and customers come in nervous and uncertain, there is no need to impress them with my filthy vernacular. Just as discussing my needs with my bike mechanic is not a necessarily a teachable moment regarding anatomical correctness. In those instances, softer words make the most sense. I will even use the words pee-pee, cookie, and front-pelvis bone if that is really what someone needs to hear to feel comfortable. My words can bend to suit any stranger. We all shift our shapes and presentations for different audiences as we navigate our own personal universe. Words, in all their power, are malleable and made to be redefined.

LOOKING FOR BLOOD

Everything was going so well that of course, something bad would happen. I was embracing my sexuality, learning about desire, and feeling safe and secure in my body. It seemed as though, through my work at Venus Envy, I had sussed out and then annihilated any and all internalized shame that I had acquired surrounding sex. I had learned that sex could be so much more than just awkward, and that there was no "right" way to do it. I had learned exactly how to make myself feel good and how to exert my sexual agency. I was feeling in control of my body, on top of the world and entirely self-certain. And then it happened.

A letter from a friend written to me during that time sums it up best: "Sometimes, you just trip and get pregnant." That is exactly how it felt. Not to remove all of my agency—I did actively make choices and consciously had a lapse in my good judgement. As we are all guilty of doing, I momentarily mistook myself as immortal (or, more topically, infertile) and threw myself full throttle into risks and danger and thoughtless moments of sex. I gave every inch of myself to those fucks, let my skin feel it all, held him inside of me and felt completely in control while choosing to relinquish all control. But still, when I took that test, when the first stick and then the second, third, and fourth each turned up their mean little plus signs, it felt just like I had tripped. That pothole came out of nowhere and sent me staggering.

And so I was pregnant. And I was going to have an abortion. I am probably the one billionth person in the world to have been in this position. Certainly I was not the first. What I experienced was not new or unique in any way. And by all means, my trials and tribulations were undoubtedly far easier than those of the people who came before me. Thanks to so many radical fighters, I did not have to use a coat hanger nor be ushered into a back alleyway. Instead, I was able to legally have an abortion in a safe hospital at no financial cost. In the grand scheme of things I was lucky. But I definitely did not feel lucky.

To say that I "staggered" is perhaps being retrospectively optimistic. It would really be more accurate to write that pregnancy was akin to being violently knocked flat on my face and losing all of my teeth. My pregnancy days were one long, cruel, meandering nightmare. It was an incredibly difficult experience, not because I did not want to have an abortion, but because it felt as though the rest of the world did not want me to. I was experiencing firsthand the ways in which patriarchal state-sanctioned structures limit the ability of people with vulvas to make choices which directly affect our bodily autonomy. It's a fucked up thing to move through and to be so viscerally affected by. You can't live through it and not be changed.

I found out for sure on September third. Which was three days after August thirtieth. Which was my twenty-fifth birthday. So maybe I should begin there. August thirtieth was my twenty-fifth birthday and on that day my period was four days late. It was four days late, that was unusual, and I was concerned; but it was my birthday, the sun was shining, and I was committed to not worrying about it just yet. I woke up early that day and went straight to the lake. It was seven a.m. and the sun was already hot on my back. I remember that I had the rocky shore all to myself, an unexpected solitude that I mistook as a good omen. Feeling hopeful about the coming year, I plunged my body into the cool water and did my own informal baptism ceremony. I rebirthed myself and came out of Long Lake one year older. As I lay drying in the sun, my phone rang. It was my mom. My grandfather had died, and I had to come home. I was on a plane within hours.

For three days, I was in Ontario at the old farmhouse. It was so hot. We were all sticky and uncomfortable, our bellies full of community casseroles and our hearts full of grief. The whole family was there, milling around. No one knew what to say or where to sit. In between meals and amidst small talk, my grandfather was buried. After the ceremony we all swapped our suits for overalls, headed out to the barn, and stayed there all night soothing tears with whisky. We laughed and cried. We retold the same familiar anecdotes to comfort one another. I don't remember much of the stories told, to be honest. I was always missing the punchline anyway. I was too busy sneaking off, ducking into bathrooms and empty bedrooms. There I would pull down my pants to examine my underwear, put my fingers inside myself, looking for blood. Each time there was nothing.

On September third, two days after burying my grandfather and three days after turning twenty-five, my period was seven days late. I got on a plane and flew back to Nova Scotia. I arrived in the city by late afternoon and went straight to the pharmacy. I picked up a pregnancy test and it felt weirdly as though my life had become a moment stolen from an early episode of Degrassi High. It felt silly and surreal, imagining that I was probably taking myself too seriously. But still, I was too nervous to open the box.

I brought the test home and put it on a shelf in my new place. On the day my grandfather had died, I had been moving into a new apartment. So now I had returned to my home feeling disjointed, unsure where things went.

I ignored the test for hours and busied myself unpacking boxes. I felt alone. The place I had just moved into was small and old. There was not enough light. It felt as though the slanted ceilings were eating me. My stuff did not seem to fit into the corners. I unloaded boxes, positioned my things, and repositioned them again. Still, nothing fit. Still, the pregnancy test sat there waiting.

I spent the whole night unpacking boxes and shuffling and reshuffling furniture. By midnight there was really only one thing left to do. With every item in its place, there were no more distractions or excuses. And so, I did it. I took the test.

This is what happens when you take a pregnancy test: you position yourself so that you can pee on this stick thing, you want to hit the stick in the right spot, but you also don't want to accidentally piss on your hand, or have bounce back and get piss all over the seat. This process seemed awkward to me, especially considering that when I pee I am already using one hand for my catheter. I decided to simplify the process and pee into a jar. I squatted down and let loose right over a mason jar which had, according to the label, contained dill pickles in 2007. Remarkably, this really did feel less awkward. Then I dipped the stick in and waited. You have to wait for two full minutes. I chose to leave the stick in the bathroom alone, with the door shut.

I thought that despite being an inanimate object, the stick needed some privacy to work its magic and ascertain my fate. While my future was being decided, I was buttering toast in the other room.

Over the next ten minutes, I dipped four sticks into that jar. The sticks, independently of one another, each arrived at the same conclusion: I was pregnant. Pregnancy tests do not give false positives. If they say yes, they mean it. And so I defied the arid vastness of my corneas. Despite the funeral and all that had happened, I still had some salt water reserves. I cried all night.

Realizing I was pregnant was heartbreaking and scary, but it was not a conundrum. It was so easy to make my decision that it almost felt as though I didn't even make one. As soon as I had had an inkling that I was pregnant I knew that if the worst were true, I would have an abortion. I had always been pro-choice, long before I had even identified as a feminist. For as far back as I could remember, it had just seemed intuitive to me that a person should be able to choose what to do with their body. No argument that operated under the thesis that someone should not be able to exert control over their own fertility had ever made much sense to me. I had always thought the opposition to abortions was a completely absurd throwback from the not-so-distant past where the complete subjugation of women went unquestioned. Denying someone access to abortion seemed comparable to denying women the right to vote: a totally wacky expression of patriarchy that insinuated that people with vulvas can not be trusted with anything. All of this meant that luckily, I did not have to work through any moral dilemma. I felt sad, scared, and alone but I was certainly certain. I called the doctor's office the very next day to book my appointment.

When you are expecting an abortion in Nova Scotia, Canada, there are multiple hoops you must jump through. Firstly, you must get an abortion referral. Secondly, you must get blood work and an ultrasound done. Thirdly, you must wait an extended period of time. Lastly, you are finally permitted to have the procedure. I went into my first hoop, the appointment for a referral, entirely unprepared for what to expect. Which is to say that I went in prepared to get what I wanted, only to find out that while I had the right to choose, I did not get to choose all that much.

I went to the health centre that day looking well-dressed and feeling powerful. As a person with a disability, I had been a patient for sixteen years at this point. What this means is that for sixteen years I had been navigating the twisted bureaucracy of the medical health system. This had afforded me a lot of time to learn how to assert myself and make sure my needs are being met. I now have a tendency to approach doctors and the medical health industry with a strong dose of skepticism. This is not because all doctors are bad. On the contrary, I have had a lot of positive experiences in my sixteen years as a patient. However, I have also had countless experiences where it felt the doctors and I were trying to assert entirely different agendas. I will come in armed with questions and they will come in expecting to give me no more than fifteen minutes. I will come in wanting recommendations for rehabilitation therapy and they will recommend drugs or injections. I do not profess to be a medical expert, but I am an expert on my own body. And when you are the patient, it is easy to feel like you are out of control, like things are being done to you, and decisions are being made for you.

After sixteen years, I have learned ways of making sure

that in my appointments, my voice is heard. I get dressed up. I speak eloquently and concisely. Essentially, I lean on my access to privilege: I use being a white, educated, middle-class cisgender[6] woman to my advantage. I went to my first appointment expecting to do just that. I knew exactly what I wanted and I wanted it very badly. I imagined that I would go in, explain the situation, and be scheduled in for an abortion a week later. Unfortunately, that is not what happened. Not at all. Having an abortion is not nearly that simple.

I entered the clinic to find the waiting room empty. I registered at the front desk and sat down on the plasticized chairs trying to look proper. I flipped through magazines, picked my nails, and tapped my toes on the stained carpet. I had been so sure that this appointment would be fast and efficient that I had scheduled myself to go into work immediately afterwards. At this point in my pregnancy I was under the impression that if I just kept really busy, working all the time, then I would be able to ignore my glaringly absent period and pretend that nothing was amiss. So I willed the doctor to hurry. I did not want to have to be still for any amount of time, avoiding all possible moments of reflection.

Eventually the nurse called me in, and thus began my hoop jumping. The first step is to go into a room to discuss your situation. A nurse asks you questions about who you are and how you feel. They ask about your menstrual period, your sexual partners, and how far along you think you may be. Then the nurse explains each of your options: to have a baby, to give a baby up for adoption, or to have what is called a therapeutic abortion, or TA. As I stumbled through our conversation and took in all of this information, I won-

---

6. I identify as a cisgender woman. This means that I identify with the gender I was assigned at birth.

dered if this was standard protocol for all pregnant people. If someone were to call the doctor and say they were pregnant and wanted to keep the baby, would they still need to discuss their options? Would the doctor suggest having an abortion? Or is it only if you are on the other side of the coin that you need to really consider these things? Either way, I knew exactly what I was doing. I had already told the nurse why I was here. But these steps were required, so I sat through them obediently, expecting this conversation would lead directly to my appointment.

When the nurse finished her explanations and I reaffirmed that I would definitely be having an abortion, I was given an information packet and ushered into a second room. This room had an examination table and I was told to remove my pants and underwear and put my feet in the cold, metal stirrups. I hoped that this would be it, something would happen on that table, and I would walk out of the clinic free of all problems. Instead, the doctor came in and put her gloves on. She explained that she was going to check and see how far along I was, and then she put her latex-clad fingers inside my vagina and pressed up against my cervix.

"Three weeks," she said as she pulled out and snapped her gloves off. I was floored. While I had assumed that I was about that far along, hearing it from someone else's mouth sank the reality in much deeper. It startled me that someone could touch my body and know that much. I wondered if others would be able to tell. Was it so obvious? Would I show? The sense of self-assuredness I had walked in with was waning and I was too baffled to ask these questions aloud. The doctor told me to put my clothes back on and return to the first room. I was a yo-yo, going back and forth. I zipped up my jeans and zipped back to the first room.

There, the same nurse as before reminded me again of my options. I again chose abortion. So the nurse explained to me what exactly would happen next: I would be referred to have an ultrasound and blood test at the hospital—to make sure that the pregnancy was not showing any complications—and then I would have "the procedure." She explained that the procedure would also take place in a private wing of the hospital. I nodded my understanding as all of this was explained. And then the nurse told me, "okay, so we will have you booked in for October fifth."

"What do you mean?" I asked. I could not imagine why I would need to come back and visit the clinic in a month's time.

"That is when you will have your TA. On October fifth, at the hospital."

"That isn't for another month!"

"That's standard. You need to be pregnant for at least eight weeks to make sure the procedure takes. By October fifth you should be at about eight and a half."

"That can't be right! No way! I work full time. I can't just hang out and be unwillingly pregnant for another four weeks."

I was panicking. I had already known I was pregnant for five days and found it to be awful. I had not experienced any symptoms yet, but just knowing that something was growing in my body, something that I did not want, was very disconcerting. My bodily autonomy was feeling wildly compromised and I was yearning for that hungry little zygote to be out of me. I could not imagine just letting it gestate in there for another twenty-eight days.

But it was going to. No matter how upset I was or how much I argued, I did not have the power to change provincial laws. The nurse kindly explained to me that there was really no way of getting around the wait period. It was just the way things were. She reassured me that pregnant women do things all the time and I would not have to put my life on pause. She said it would be unlikely that I would even experience any symptoms. "You'll be fine," she said.

I left the clinic feeling defeated and angry. It seemed the State was punishing me. I knew that in other provinces there was not such a lengthy wait time. I had friends who had had abortions in Toronto and they had been able to have the procedure within a week of finding out. And I knew other people who had gotten pregnant on the West Coast and had had access to medical abortions, where they did not have to wait, or be hospitalized, but had instead taken an oral pill. This East Coast experience was feeling comparatively draconian.

I was sure the wait time was in part practical. With only one hospital serving most of the province and Prince Edward Island, I imagined a long list of people were waiting and I was just put into the queue. But I also felt suspiciously like I was being patronized too. These laws seemed like a measure intended to make us all reflect on our sins and feel guilty. It felt like the eight weeks were a reminder that we were on a short leash, that we weren't really in control at all. At the end of the day, I was just another slutty woman who had erred and would have to deal with the consequences. It all felt so paternalistic. I knew exactly who I was and what I wanted. As an adult I had the tools to understand that actions have consequences. I knew about remorse and I also knew how to forgive myself. I definitely did not need the Law to teach me these lessons.

I went into my wait time kicking up against it. I felt so angry that I thought I would surely be angry for the full four weeks. But that didn't happen. Getting pregnant was a lesson in many things, not the least of which was learning that everything I expect to happen may very well not happen. As I waited there in my pregnancy, all my anger fizzled into shame. The futility of raging at a system that you are powerless to rectify is extremely disheartening. In the face of it my anger withered. I was too tired to be anything other than tired. Being pregnant zapped everything out of me. So instead of being righteous and raging, my pregnancy was full of shame and exhaustion. I walked into it sure of myself and walked out deflated. The silence around abortion, paired with the time I spent waiting, made me doubt myself and feel I had done something wrong. I felt completely ashamed of myself for finding myself pregnant and without a partner. Shunned, shamed, and silenced—all the bad Ss.

Your body may go through a lot of different things during the first nine weeks of pregnancy. I do not profess to know all of them, but I can tell you what I felt. I know it isn't technically an emotion, but one of the primary things I felt was hunger. I could eat absolutely everything, except vegetables. If it was a carb and within five feet of me you could expect it to be in my mouth. With renewed vigor, I loved macaroni and cheese, pasta, and cereal. I could eat an entire loaf of sourdough for breakfast. Paired with this new hunger was a heightened sense of smell. For real, pregnant people develop some serious nose-strength. While it is probably some evolutionary by-product intended to help sniff out life-threatening predators, I used to it to suss out sweets. I followed my nose to every cake, cookie, and crumpet in the city and promptly shoved them into my pie-hole.

When I wasn't eating, I was fast asleep. It felt like I could sleep forever. Fourteen hours a night became my norm and

I would still wake up tired in the morning. I would drag my body to work and then back to my bed. So much for keeping busy and distracting myself—doing anything, other than what was absolutely necessary, seemed impossible.

There were so many things that signaled that my body was no longer all my own. My breasts swelled and felt misshapen. My vulva smelled strong and musky. (I spent the duration of my pregnancy with my legs crossed, irrationally afraid that if I should open them, someone would smell my fertility). The smell of coffee and cigarettes, my two most favoured vices, became abhorrent. The mornings became a time when I would vomit. The nights became a time when I would cry. The afternoons could not be predicted. I was completely out of control.

I spent a lot of that time alone. We are taught not to speak about abortions and I followed the rules. When people asked how I was doing, I would smile, and nod, and speak of the weather. I would lie. How can one be honest? Should I have answered that I was pregnant? It was strange and burdensome to be holding on to this secret. I have never held secrets. My mouth is a sieve that lets everything through. But I did not think I could talk about this one thing. So it stayed secret and I stayed isolated, as secrets will do. They turn you into a lonely island.

And then October fifth came and suddenly it was all over, just like that.

The night before my abortion it rained and rained. I repainted my walls, replacing the white emptiness with Egyptian Sunrise—a warm orange. It had felt like I ought to either paint my walls or shave my head, do something outward to mark my massive internal shift. Vanity has forever barred head shaving as an option for me, so the walls were all that was left. When I woke up on October fifth, it was to the smell of paint drying on sticky walls.

It was five thirty a.m. and the sky was still dark and sunless. Two friends and I crowded into my car. I lay down in the back seat. My abortion was unfortunately timed to occur during the Forty Days for Life protests, forty days every year during which anti-abortion activists stand outside of hospitals and clinics across North America, shaming those of us who have had to make the difficult choice to terminate a pregnancy. It is a truly detestable vigil they hold, mourning the deaths of "babies" without any consideration for the pain that those of us who are pregnant may be experiencing, and disregarding our right to choose what happens to our bodies. Predictably, the protests are populated primarily by old, cisgender white men. Men with bodies that have never been pregnant, with bodies that have never had their reproductive rights denied. I lay down in my back seat as we drove up to the City Hospital not to protect myself from their judging eyes but to protect them from my forceful fists. Without a doubt, if I were to have looked at them right then, with all the pain I was holding and all the exhaustion I was feeling, I would have let loose. Nothing could have held me back. I would have missed my abortion appointment that I had been waiting so long for if only to fight them, if only to show them the depths of my anger, if only to lay all of my wrath on their old, bigoted bones. I could have left it there with them, my rage and my hurt and my fury, and walked away lighter. But instead, I ducked down in my back seat and saved my strength for myself. My abortion was more important.

Inside the hospital, I was separated from my friends and led through a strange fluorescent maze. The abortion division, or whatever it is called, is laid out at the end of a windowless maze of tunnels to protect the staff. Performing abortions was dangerous, and sometimes still is, and so the doctors and the nurses and those of us who are pregnant are all hidden from the outside world. My friends were sent to one waiting room and I was brought through the maze to another. I waited with other women for a couple of hours. One of us would be called up, led away, and would not come back. Again, I bit my nails. Again, I pretended to read the magazines. Eventually, it was my turn.

"Kaleigh Trace."

I stood up, solemn. I followed the nurse into another room and was given a locker. I took off all of my clothes and put on a long, green gown, then progressed into a third room where I was offered drugs.

"Opiates, Ativan, or nothing at all?" the nurse asked.

Part of me wanted to choose nothing at all. This was going to be one of the biggest moments of my life and I wanted to experience it soberly, without a clouded mind or a subdued heart. But as I weighed my decision, I realized my fingertips were caked in blood because I has bitten my nails down to the quick. I noticed that my knees were shaking, and I was holding on to the wall for support. It was clear that I did not quite have my shit together. So, I obediently took the small paper cup of Ativan and swallowed.

Shortly thereafter I was led into the fourth and final room. Again, just like during my very first appointment, I was presented with cold metal stirrups to place my feet in. I lay down on the bed cloaked in crinkly paper and got into position. Above me three fluorescent bulbs beamed down and hurt my eyes. I began to cry, afraid that I would just lay in that room alone while a machine performed some painful procedure. I had no idea what to expect, but the white walls and the smell of disinfectant were not reassuring. Luckily, that is not how abortions are performed. It is not a wordless operation acted out by inanimate, cold, beeping machinery. For something so painful, it was an event that felt deeply human and tender.

A nurse came in and held my hand and spoke to me through it all. She encouraged me to look into her eyes and not down at the doctor between my legs. She issued me reassurances about my choice, about my strength, about being a good woman. Throughout all of it she never let go of my hands, even when the vacuuming began and I squeezed so hard that I thought I heard her fingers crack. She squeezed back, and stroked my hair, and kept murmuring to me as the doctor moved in and out of the room, brusquely explaining what was happening. In total, the procedure itself must have taken less than ten minutes. Just like that, my womb was emptied and my body was all mine again.

That same nurse put me in a chair and wheeled me into the recovery room where I was given milk and cookies and a snack pack of cheese and crackers. The food, in its neat packaging and tiny portions, felt oddly like treats provided to children on lunch break. Throughout all of this, I could not stop sobbing. I slobbered into the cheese and crackers. I swallowed the snacks like they were medicine, tasting nothing but my own mucus. The nurse stayed with me as I ate, and cried, and bled onto my gown. It was not a glamorous moment. It did not matter. No one asked me why I was crying or told me to stop. It was a place accustomed to tears and so I gave in to them fully.

Half an hour later, I was with my friends again, ready to go back out into the world. I ducked down in my backseat and we went out the way we had come in, as though nothing had changed, though everything had.

It all happened just like that. One morning it was over. Only it wasn't really over. I was not pregnant anymore, but there was still an emotional hangover to work through. I did that the only way I knew how—by talking. When I was finished using my energy being pregnant, I began using my energy to talk about it. I realized that I had been silent because I had absorbed a falsely constructed sense of shame that I wanted to expel.

I refuse to believe that I was wrong for having an abortion. Instead, I think I was brave, and I am proud of myself and all of us who have moved through that experience. We are strong and we are many. Abortions are not all that rare so it is almost remarkable that they are still talked about in hushed voices. I do not want to hush my voice.

The more I talk about my experience, the more it transforms from MY ABORTION into my abortion, something I lived through but that does not define me. Each word that leaves my mouth takes with it some weight from off my shoulders. And so I cannot stop talking about it. I have to talk and talk and talk. Not only because talking is what I do, but because talking is the only way I can rectify having once held such a secret. I want to use words to deconstruct old ideas. I want to use words to lay new foundations for new attitudes, ones that are more kind. I want to learn from my experience and share it so we can all learn. I want for others who may have an abortion to be able to walk into it with their heads up and their hearts strong and their mouths wide open, shouting their own words and stories out into the world. Together, our shared stories can coalesce and become a force, a force so strong that no one can stop us. And we will talk and we will talk and we will talk and we will be unstoppable.

(NOT) MOVING LIKE A DYKE/ (ALWAYS) DRESSING LIKE A FEMME

I am a queer, disabled woman. There. I said it. It was obvious, I know, but it is important for me to say it all the same. Queer, disabled woman. I say it with complete certainty. But this has taken a long, long time. I've been peeling those labels on and off my chest for nineteen years. I've rearranged them (queer woman with a disability), altered them (bi-curious dis/abled woman), and added to them (queer, disabled, sex-positive, femme, cisgender woman, for example). Ultimately, queer, disabled woman feels best (for right now).

I was in my car accident in 1995. This is when I sustained my spinal cord injury which effectively led me to being a person with a disability. Since that time I have had my swaying legs, my indomitable bladder, and my chronic pain. Since that time, the world has looked at me as I've teetered through my life and called me disabled—I definitely do not live up to an able-bodied norm. I am not normal.

I initially did not even *like* this truth, let alone love it as I do now. As a kid I completely rejected that label. I could see no reason for wanting to embrace a word that seemed synonymous with weaker, lesser than, and unattractive. Like most kids, all I wanted was to fit in. So I learned quickly how to hide and disregard my differences. I wore clothing and shoes that I hoped would draw attention away from my leg braces. At recess and in gym glass I would "run" around with the other kids, stumbling after them with my quad canes as support. I would make an effort at soccer, tree-climbing, and dodge ball. I would laugh off all my trips and falls. I would do absolutely anything to be just like everyone else.

Predictably, this drive to attain regularity only grew as I entered high school—the homogenizing, clone-producing factory that it is. As soon as I set foot in the ninth grade, I knew that there was no way I wanted to be noticed as "different." I wanted popularity, boyfriends, and all of those good times I had seen in *Dazed and Confused*, *Empire Records*, and *She's All That*. I wanted to live the Teen Dream.

The first shaky step to the end goal was to stop using my cane. Up until this point my mother had been painstakingly painting my canes to match my outfits: one was baby-doll pink with glitter, and another was blue with little white clouds spread out across it. This no longer mattered to me. I was sure that having a "walking aid" would immediately draw attention to me and prohibit me from getting a date. In fact, I was convinced my eighth-grade boyfriend had dumped me because his older brother had teased him for dating the "disabled girl." It was crucial to me that this not happen again. So I would use my cane to get on the bus and then hide it in my locker all day. When I was strong enough, I stopped using it altogether. I would risk any tumble to not have it. I was certain that without it, I was passing as normal and desirable.

Throughout my high school years, I loped around with a wobble at every field party, barn party, and tailgate party. No matter how rocky and uneven the terrain, I would go where everyone else was going and do what everyone else was doing.

I would get shit-faced, hit the bong, jump into dark, rocky quarries, and do whatever it took to fit in. For the most part, I was happy. It felt like I was living the life I had watched in the movies. I had boyfriends, nice clothes and I went to parties. My disability did not go unnoticed, but I was able to access enough spaces to make it so that it seemed to not affect me. I could do almost everything the other kids did. I never once called myself disabled. I was just like everyone else. And no matter how much my feet hurt or my back ached at the end of the night, I always thought it was worth it.

Then the day came that I decided to leave small town Ontario for the big, bad, and much more challenging Real World. The day that I arrived in Halifax, Nova Scotia was the day that things began to change. I was in a new place without my old station wagon to get me around nor my little brother to carry my book bag. I was at a new university with a big maze of a campus and many old buildings with multiple flights of stairs. I was living in a residence that was full of nondisabled party animals who always wanted to walk fast and drunkenly to the bar downtown. I was trying to ride city buses that did not allow you to stop for a pee break. Everything was suddenly a million times more difficult. The conceptual fallacy that I had been embracing for years was facing its reckoning: I was not like everybody else.

This recognition dawned on me pretty quickly, especially considering how long I had been locking it in an attic. Within six months of leaving home I began calling myself "a person with a disability." The facts were too clear to ignore: I could not make it to class on time, could not walk as fast my friends, and did not want to ride the city bus for fear of peeing my pants. So, like any stranger in a new place, I was given the option to reinvent myself, and I chose to move in a more honest direction. I slowly turned to disability and I looked at it, head on. What I found upon my examination was some serious ableism and self-hate.

I started reading a whole lot of disability theory and was seeking out disability pop culture at this point. As I learned more and more, I realized that denying my identity and not calling myself disabled was an ableist manifestation. I had bought into the idea that able-bodied people were more valuable than those who are disabled, and I was upholding that dangerous delusion by not embracing my true self. As I read critical disability theorists, such as Catherine Frazee and Mia Mingus, I slowly but surely undid some of the misunderstood knots I had tied around my heart. I slowly but surely looked at my crooked feet and fell in love with them. I slowly but surely grew more comfortable asking for help. I began to love myself in my entirety. I began to reclaim what it meant for me to have a spinal cord injury. I began to love calling myself disabled. I no longer wanted to reproduce ableist oppression by denying my identity. I no longer wanted to try to be something I was not.

Within the disabled community I embody a lot of privilege. I can access all sorts of spaces. I can stand upright in front of a room of people and have them listen to my loud voice. This privilege must be noted. Disability is so broad and ableism can affect us in so many different ways. The way that I experience disability has meant that I lived without fully recognizing it for a long time. And so the route I took to arrive at lovingly calling myself disabled was a long and winding one. I had to deconstruct and then rebuild so much of what I thought was true. I had to recognize the fucked up shit I had ignorantly done, and had to rework so much of my own damaging beliefs. I am still working on all of this.

In many ways I have not yet "arrived" anywhere. While I proudly call myself a disabled woman, there is still so much I am learning and there are so many ways in which I am still growing.

Coming to call myself queer has been a similarly serpentine path. It was not straightforward nor immediate. I flirted with queer for years. For most of my life I had been eyeing it's broad shoulders and wondering if I would fit into its plaid shirts.

I grew up surrounded by lesbians. I'm not exaggerating. They were literally everywhere. They lived in my basement and attended all my family parties. Gay women essentially were my family parties. I come from one big, noisy, pretty gay matriarchy. My mother has fourteen siblings, and those fourteen siblings collectively birthed forty-one blonde-haired, blue-eyed, round-bottomed babies. Most of those babies were girls (twenty-six, to be exact) and all of those girls learned quickly how to be loud.

My mother and her sisters have always ruled the roost. If you were to ask a Lalonde, "who's the boss?" my mother and each of her sisters would answer that they are. They are women in control, and they taught their daughters that skill, or maybe we all just contracted it by osmosis. Lalonde girls are always in charge, they tell the most vulgar jokes, and they have a penchant for being queerer than a two dollar bill. A whole slew of my cousins are bona fide, brilliant gay women.

Within this matriarchal structure, I was the thirty-sixth little bundle of fatty, pink flesh rolls to be popped out. This means that I have always been one of the youngest of the pack. I have spent the duration of my life thus far following around my older, smarter, cooler cousins. I wore Converse sneakers because they wore Converse sneakers, I played tee-ball because they played tee-ball and I listened to Prince because they listened to Prince. My identity has essentially always just been one epic act of mimicry. So being queer has always been an option, if not even an inevitability for me. As a kid I had never thought of it as a particularly strange, scary, or dangerous identity to embrace. And still it took me years to arrive here, at calling myself by its name.

Perhaps predictably, my desires started to veer off the straight and narrow path shortly after beginning work at Venus Envy. I don't think it was Venus Envy exactly that made me gay, but rather, being surrounded by an almost entirely queer staff every day helped suss out and fertilize those deeply-rooted queer feelings. Within six months of working there, my fantasies were getting all jumbled up and confused. I started looking at everyone a little differently. I would cock my head at every queer-looking person who would walk into the shop and wonder if I was attracted to them or if I just wanted to be them. At first I thought I was maybe just homesick for my big, lesbian family and was feeling drawn to dykes on account of that. I could not quite figure it out.

And then came my first Big Gay Crush. I became obsessed with a woman named Jane who was so good-looking she'd get my panties wet just looking at her. We met at a potluck of a friend of a friend. She was just passing through town and had nowhere to stay. By the end of our five minute, introductory conversation, I selflessly offered to share my bed with her. She slurped a noodle from her bowl of vegan pad thai, shrugged her shoulders, and said, "sure."

For weeks, she stayed with me, and I would lie beside her at night, literally shaking. Her back to me, I would look at the curve of her back and will myself not to touch her. Even being near her would sometimes make me want to puke. My attraction was so painfully visceral that for a short time I was truly convinced not that I was gay, but that I had the stomach flu. It was raw and all-consuming. It was also a totally unsustainable emotional state to live in. I had to tell her. So, one night I got drunk at the gay bar and confessed my baby-gay, butterfly feelings.

"Listen, we need to talk about what's going on here. I think we should kiss," I declared both boldly and sloppily, as my drink sloshed around in my cup.

Jane looked at me with pity, explained that "straight girls weren't her type," and left town a few days later.

That was it. She was gone as fast as she had come, and I was one crushed puppy. With Jane's blunt rejection and departure, my gay feelings faded. I assumed that she was probably right. For an embarrassingly long time, I had believed that queer people could somehow sense their own kind, as if everyone was equipped with a gay divining rod. I trusted Jane's judgement of me. I must be straight. All the signs pointed that way. For instance, I wore dresses. In my childhood I had been obsessed with Barbies, ponies, and princesses. I loved lipstick and nail polish. I listened to folky indie pop. In no way did I match up to the image of queer that I had come to understand through watching my cousins and my co-workers. My floral-patterned blouses felt more comfortable than button-down flannels. I did not know how to build anything. I did not have that confident swagger I had observed in so many masculine of centre folks I knew. In no way did I move like a dyke. In every way I always dressed like a femme.

I have learned everything from books. So, post-Jane and

reeling from my crush, I turned to queer theory. I read *Brazen Femme*, *Whipping Girl*, and *Persistence*. I looked for versions of me in these books. I wanted to learn about expressions of queerness that looked different from those I had always known. I wanted to hear from the experts. Could I be queer? Did it still count if I had such long hair? (You may think this hang up on hair is absurd, but queer haircuts are an institution. Hair can be one of the most important markers). As I read more and more and more and found diverse portrayals of queerness and femininity, I began to question why it was exactly that I was so reluctant to call myself queer.

For a long time I had assumed that the way that I looked, coupled with my attraction to masculinity, implied an obvious straightness. Plus, I knew so many powerful people who had struggled and fought for the label queer that I did not want to misuse it. I thought I had not wanted to call myself queer out of a concern of appropriation, not wanting to take on an identity that was not rightfully mine. But perhaps I had been denying my queerness for reasons similar to those I had had when denying my disability. It seemed I had some internalized femmephobia that I had to work through. I had unconsciously limited gay women to looking a very particular way, a way that I just did not look. I had so strongly come to believe that queer could only mean a few things that I had been overlooking the importance of queering femininity. I had not understood that I could wear my curls long and my skirts short with a brazen toughness that had nothing to do with heternormativity. Queer could look my way too.

Much like with disability, I came to queer through an undoing. I undressed the grey pantsuit of my femmephobia and instead put on a sparkly, hot pink mini skirt. Now, I know that queer fits. Queer makes space for my criss-crossing legs, my flaming-red lipstick, and my big hair. In queerness I can have a kind of sex that denies any kind of trajectory or framework, a kind of sex that allows for the complexities of disability and gender. Queer leans left with my politics and fits right between my legs. I am a disabled, queer femme, and I love queer bodies.

The labels queer and disabled fit well together and I am honoured to hold them both. They fit together because they both involve resistance. Resistance against those tired ideas of what and how one should be, resistance against presumed and ill-fitting "truths" about the world. In this resistance, both of these words work to create a much-needed space. Space for bodies to be valued in and of themselves, space for beauty and love to be redefined.

THE MOMENT AT WHICH ONE HAS GONE TOO FAR

There comes a time when you worry that you have crossed your own boundaries. You shove your foot so far in your mouth that you think you may have swallowed it. You can almost feel it kicking around down there in your guts. Personally, I do not experience this all that often. My boundaries are so far gone that they are nearly non-existent. Peeing on that man really decimated them years ago and I just never got around to building them back up. However, despite their lack of substance, they are still there. When I ram up against them I am always shocked, taken aback by the discovery that I still got 'em. Most recently a little mishap with the written word wound me up there—pressed up against those long-forgotten brick walls of my personal comfort zone.

It all began with a bout of unsatisfactory sex. I was stuck in one. Nobody was knocking on my door and my own hands weren't getting the job done right, either. I had just experienced my first big, bad, gay heartbreak and I was convinced that I would never have sex with another person again. You know that thing that happens when you try to masturbate but instead wind up crying on your bed, naked and alone and thinking about your eternal future of loneliness, misery, and too many cats? I did that. A lot. It is an extremely pathetic position to be in and one I hope not to revisit. I mean, I suppose it's good that it happened because "whatever doesn't kill you only makes you stronger" and yadda-yadda-yadda, but whatever. I still think that tired consolation is trite and I would prefer to not contort myself into the confines of romance-related self-pity ever again.

Anyway, the point is that I wasn't having sex at all, ever, and was instead spending most of my time being sad and eating dairy products. My eyes were looking all red and bulgy all the time and I was losing weight. My nose was on auto-drip. After crying at work for the fifth time, I decided that something had to be done. In an attempt to ease my shattered little heart and stem the dry spell, I turned to erotica. Watching porn has never really done it for me, even radical queer porn. My attention span for TV is just too short. But I optimistically hoped that reading erotica would be different. I borrowed a bunch of books from the shop, grabbed a fresh bottle of lube, and went home to try and get down.

My hopes were misplaced. My attempts were made in vain. Reading erotic literature had the opposite effect on my lack of libido. If there had been any juices there to begin with, they would have dried up. Essentially, the erotica was abhorrent. I may be no perfect specimen of an author myself, but seriously, you should have seen this stuff. It was bad. Real bad. In straight erotica, the women were always biting their lips while the men were unconsciously flexing their rippling biceps. If it was lesbian erotica I was reading, these same predictable roles were being reproduced with "butch and femme" replacing "man and woman." Everything felt repetitive and done before. It was all passive feminine characters and more masculine domineering ones. It was all nondisabled, cisgender, white people. It was all penetration and coming, multiple orgasms and seamless sex. None of it reminded me of me. I am so often looking for myself in sexual imagery, for people like me: people who have different bodies and abilities, who make mistakes and laugh at inopportune moments. And so often I come up empty-handed, wanting more.

I read all this erotica, I didn't get off, and I found myself getting more and more frustrated. I was surrounded by sex toys, candles, and a near empty bottle of whisky, and I was still not even close to coming. All my reading and drinking had just left me wasted and worked up in all the wrong ways. So, in a spell of drunken sexlessness, I decided I would take matters into my own hands. I resolved that if you wanted something done right you have to do it yourself. I would just have to write my own erotica featuring a person with a disability. Easy. I pulled out my laptop and in half an hour it was done. Feeling righteous and victorious, I posted it online and passed out in my clothes on top of my bed sheets.

The things that I had not considered when making this rash decision are as follows:

1. My mother, my grandmother, my aunts, and my cousins follow me on the internet.
2. When a disabled woman writes a piece of erotica about a disabled woman, most people who read it are going to assume the sex represented is the kind of sex she is having.
3. The internet is a big, bad black hole where things spread faster than HPV.

When I woke up the next morning, I found that my blog post had been read by 782 people overnight. There was a stern voicemail on my answering machine from my mother, reminding me that my grandmother is quite proficient at using the internet. When I went outside, I felt like I was receiving nothing but curious glances from strangers and friends alike. When doing my shopping at the market that weekend, a man I only vaguely knew nonchalantly whispered to me that he was "interested in power play." Later that same night I went to a dance party and received not one but three different sexy propositions (suffice it to say the dry spell ended then and there).

All in all, it was a pretty strange experience. It felt like I had unintentionally opened my bedroom door to nearly eight hundred strangers, and they had all watched me writhing around naked and sweaty. And to be entirely honest, I was fully embarrassed and drowning in self-doubt. I began wondering why I keep using public forums as a place to unload my personal opinions. Couldn't I just get a fucking diary already? What is wrong with me? I almost wanted to undo my drunken literary mistakes, despite the positive attention it had garnered.

Luckily, the joy of finally having sex again trumped the sheepishness I was feeling about being such a sexualized extrovert. I chose to not remove my smutty blog post. Instead I thought critically about why I was feeling so bashful anyway. All sorts of people (porn stars, writers, etc.) expose facets of their sexuality all the time. Who am I to feel embarrassed? Plus, I remembered, if my aim in writing that piece of erotica was to further the representation of people with disabilities in sexual settings, than I had actually achieved my goal just fine. People had seemingly read it and liked it.

I now knew of at least one piece of erotica that involved a body like mine. Everything was actually a success, and feeling embarrassed about it all was just some useless hang-up remaining from my more private past. Looking back, I can embrace that writing that erotica had felt damn good.

And so here it is again, that very piece of dirty smut. If you think you may have hit a personal boundary and stepped outside of your comfort zone, you might as well step out of it again.

FUCK ME ANYWHERE

The bar was hot and crowded. Bodies pressed against bodies, beats pressed against ear drums, and all I wanted was for them to press me against the wall. I wanted to be held up and fucked. I wanted their hands to push against me so hard that they would leave marks. That feeling of being held up, thrown around, pressed on, and pried at until I am completely pliable—that's what I wanted more than anything.

"I need to go to the bathroom," I yelled up at them. The music carried my quiet voice away and so I propelled myself forward, my wheels gently knocking their ankles so that they stumbled back a little, their ass falling against me. They were straddling my chair now, their weight on top of me, and even this contact, having their sweaty back pressed against my chest, our bodies still fully clothed, felt like too much. I wanted it so bad.

"I need to go to the bathroom," I said again, and to make my point clear, I pulled their earlobe into my mouth, drawing the soft skin between my sharp teeth.

They looked at me, obediently. They were as ready as I was.

People cleared a path for us as we went deeper into the bar. We reached our destination and entered the one-room wheelchair bathroom together. In situations like this, I sometimes wonder what people are thinking. Do they think my lover is only my assistant, helping me to transfer onto the toilet? Does anyone suspect that what we do in these private places and darkened corners is not always about my disability, but is most often just about pure pleasure? We are usually just fucking each other in these bathrooms, a thin wall separating us from the public. The people at the party outside have no idea what kind of highs we are reaching in these stolen moments, and their ignorance just makes me wetter.

We were alone together in the grimy room and I wanted everything. I wanted it all, and all at once. I wanted them in my mouth, wanted them to cram their fingers down my throat with one hand while their other hand reached inside me. I wanted to feel full of them.

But I made myself wait.

Sweat had dripped down and pooled in my clavicle. "Lick it," I told them, and their rough tongue complied, scratching against my skin, making my cunt wet.

"Take my shirt off," and the silk was being pulled up over my head, exposing my tits to the hot, muggy air. My nipples were already hard, and they bent over me, pulling first one and then the other into their mouth.

"Now, put me..." I began, but they interrupted.

"No, my turn," they said.

We have this problem, the two of us. Two controlling people wanting to call all the shots, wanting to fuck and be fucked exactly the way we want, wanting to say how it's going to be. But sometimes I like being told what to do as much as I like doing the telling.

They didn't tell me what to do, but instead, made me do it, putting my body exactly where they wanted it, controlling me, contorting me. They lifted me out of my chair and I was up against the wall. I held onto the bars, supporting myself with my arms. I can do this, but they know it makes me tired. They know that when they have me here like this, up against the wall and waiting, that they better fuck me and they better fuck me hard and fast until I am coming all over them, falling into their arms with the intensity of it all.

With one hand they pulled my hair, wrapping it tightly around their fist so my head was pulled to the side, exposing my neck for their teeth to bite into. With the other hand they pulled off my skirt. Their fingers slipped down and pressed against the soft cotton of my underwear. I could feel my clit throbbing beneath their touch. They must have felt it too, my body pulsing against them, and so they eased their fingers around my thong and against my lips.

They started gently, stroking me, teasing me.

They knew I wanted them inside me, that I was impatient and waiting and aching for it, but they wouldn't give in right away. They kept it up, those subtle strokes, up and down, up and down, until I was so wet I was dripping on their fingers. My thighs were damp with my own juice and still they would not draw me open, would not reach deeper.

I couldn't take it.

"Baby," I said. "Baby, fuck me."

"Now?" they asked.

"Right now."

"Right, right now?"

"NOW."

"And if I don't?"

"You have to."

"I have to?"

"Yeah…"

"Tell me what you want."

"I want you to fuck me hard. I want you inside me up to your wrist."

"And what's the magic word?"

"NOW!"

They acquiesced. Part of them wanted me there all night, pressed against them and begging, but they also wanted to please me.

I felt their hand move my lips open. Their rough thumb stroked my clit, while their long, beautiful fingers reached down inside me. One finger, then two, then three, were in my pussy, circling. My cunt clenched around their digits. I wanted to swallow them up, wanted them never to leave my body.

My clit got harder and harder under their

thumb. I know that they love this, love feeling how much my body wants them. And as they rubbed my clit, over and over, I expanded to take them in. My slit got wider and wider and they slid all of themselves into me. Their wrist bone pressed up against my swollen sex. It felt like everything was happening all at once. My neck was in their mouth, my nipple twisted in between their fingers, my clit pressed under their thumb, and my whole body riding their hand as it thrust into me, deeper and deeper. We moved together. I propelled myself against their body, forcing them further into me, driving them faster, and making them my own. They pressed harder and harder against my G-spot, working me. They are rough with me but I can take it. Can take it and then some.

I began to tremble. My knees buckled. And then I crumbled. It felt too good. I felt too much. I couldn't stand any more. I fell forward, my soft tits pressed against their hard chest, while I gushed all over them. I came, and came, and it felt like I wouldn't stop coming, my whole body convulsing against theirs. My hair in their mouth, their neck against my lips, my cream wetting both of us, our sweat intermingled.

Finally, they stopped. They pulled out of me, and we stared at each other, not wanting to move, not wanting to end it.

Until there was a knock at the door.

They hurriedly helped me dress. In these moments I love their range of touch. That they can fuck me hard and fast, so good that it hurts, and then gently pull my shirt over my arms, zip my zipper, and put me into my chair.

We left the bathroom, cheeks flushed. The people outside smiled at us politely. I smiled back. I imagine they thought "what a trooper!" Often that's what people are thinking when they smile at me in a particular way. They don't know that my return grin means so much more, that I am laughing at them. They are about to use a bathroom that I just flooded with my come, that smells like my sex.

Suckers.

THE TALE OF THE WOODEN DICKS

I am always half asleep at the Saturday morning Farmers' Market. Blurry-eyed, I fondle the bags of greens and boxes of berries. My breath is bad and crud is all caught up in my tear ducts. I have most likely just rolled out of bed and wiggled into the night-before-jeans to make my way downtown. Often Friday night's mascara and lipstick remain smeared across my cheeks and stale cigarette smoke emanates from my hair. In short, I am not entirely alert on Saturday mornings. But I get up and roll downtown all the same, no matter the conditions. This is in large part out of habit. I have been going to the Market for nearly a decade now. By this point, my limbs move in that direction voluntarily.

The Wood-Working Woman has been there since the beginning. Enter into the atrium of the big brick brewery that houses the Farmers' Market and you will find her there, laughing. She has been the first person I see on Saturday mornings for the last nine years. A table full of beautifully carved cutting boards, smoothed salad bowls, and ornate soup spoons stand in front of her. Every weekend she drives in from the South Shore to sell them. You'd think she'd be tired and cranky, having gotten up at three-thirty a.m. for her commute. But no, she is ceaselessly loud and friendly. She yells a booming hello to me every week, whether or not I want to talk. Her big, red face juts out smiling over her wares, welcoming me to the day. She reminds me of both my mother and my bowel movements. Like my mother, she is unselfconsciously beautiful and friendly. Like my shits, she is consistent, and experiencing her feels really positive.

Considering this relationship spans nine years, our exchanges have become predictable. We say our how-do-you-do's. We talk of the weather. I am hungry. She is caffeinated. We speak briefly, we smile, I move on. Always, it has gone this way. Or at least almost always, with the exception of one very significant deviation.

This digression from the norm happened on a morning that felt like any other. It was late July and oh so hot. I was sticky with sweat as I pulled open the heavy door to the market and sardined myself in with the mass of grocery shoppers and tourists. If I remember correctly, I was actually sticky with sweat that whole summer long without end. It was the summer of 2009, the summer of repetitive heat waves, and the summer I worked two jobs. I would spend mornings slinging coffee for wealthy old people who would walk with entitlement off of cruise ships and demand a cappuccino. Come the afternoon, I would change clothes and hobble in the heat up the hill to Venus Envy. From noon until evening I slung not beverages but dildos, usually to a much nicer crowd.

But this Saturday was my day off, so I was sweaty but not working, groggy but not cranky, ready to eat and drink coffee and sit out back in the summer heat with my friends and do the weekend crossword. I eased my way deeper into the market, wiggling around older folks and baby carriages.

As I reached the Wood-Working Woman, I found myself inadvertently jammed up against her table, momentarily trapped by the meandering crowd. I looked up and there she was, coffee in hand and smile on face.

"HI SWEETHEART, HOW YOU DOING?" she shouted at me cheerfully.

"Oh, just fine, same old," I replied. "How are you doing?"

"Well, I'm not complaining, but mostly because nobody'd listen."

"Fair enough," I smiled, as she laughed at her own oft-repeated joke.

"But I will say it has been too damned hot out there," she proceeded to complain happily.

I agreed, we both nodded our mutual understanding, and on a typical day, this would have been the point at which I moved on. But the mass of people had not shifted and I was still trapped in one place, specifically in the place directly in front of her. It was necessary for our predictable, repetitious exchange to be advanced.

"So, what do you do?" The Wood-Working Woman asked pleasantly.

"Grmm, a book store," I mumbled.

Considering I had just started my job at the sex shop and I had not yet figured out how exactly to introduce my work. It would not be accurate to say that I was embarrassed, but I was often concerned that I would unintentionally make other people embarrassed. I could not yet gauge what was socially acceptable to say and what was not. So if someone seemed like an elder whom I should respect, or a person who was not comfortable talking about sex, I would use the old book store euphemism. It was not a lie exactly, just an omission. Not knowing much about the Wood-Working

Woman, book store seemed like the safest bet.

"Oh, that is a nice job for a nice sweetheart like you. Which one?" she dug deeper.

"Downtown." I averted my eyes.

"Which one downtown?"

"Barrington Street." I answered begrudgingly. My cheeks were turning a bright pink.

"JWD Books?" She guessed.

"Nope."

"United Books?"

The questions would not stop.

"No. Uh. No. Uh. Venus Envy." I gave in and told her. I was trapped.

I looked up to notice that her eyes had lit up and she was smiling broadly. Not the predicted reaction. She threw her head back laughing. I offered a shrug. She reached her hands down, bending her knees and wordlessly sifting through her boxes of supplies. At the same time the crowd closed in around me and I was shoved up closer, my hips pressed hard against the table. And then the next thing I knew there was two gigantic wooden penises being wielded wildly around my face.

"LOOK AT THESE FELLAS!" she said, in case I had somehow not noticed them.

"I've been making these for years! They are very popular down where I'm from. Big sellers. I keep 'em under wraps in the city here for the children's sake. Gotta know a magic word to see 'em. I think they'd be a big hit though, at a store like yours. They shine up right nice and they are completely seamless. I carve 'em all by hand—big ones, small ones, little ones for your bum too."

I did not know what to say. I stared at the shining wooden

cocks in silence.

"Well, whadda'ya think, sweetheart? Could they do well up here? This is the kinda thing you're dealin' with, isn't it?"

"Yeah, I mean, uh, yeah, that's, uh, that is my job. I, uh, I just, I, um, didn't expect you to be in this line of...uh... work," I explained. I still had not had a coffee. And I was flabbergasted.

"Hmph," she grunted, eyebrows raised. "You didn't think it was just you young city things who were up for a little fun, did ya?"

She had me. I had not presumed the South Shore of Nova Scotia to be a hotbed for wooden dildos. Clearly, I had misjudged.

She continued to extoll the virtues of wooden dongs for the next five minutes while I tried to politely absorb the things she was saying. My brain had been jolted awake by the double dicks in the face, but I was still completely unsure of how to respond. Clearly my concerns about making people uncomfortable had been pretty off mark, at least in this instance. Was everyone so laissez-faire about sex? Were my feelings of shyness and uncertainty about my new job signs of my supreme naivety?

When she finally finished, I walked away pleasantly baffled. It was fair to say my admiration for the Wood-Working Woman had quadrupled. Making your own dildos is a pretty rad move, even if I did think it was rather eccentric at the time. While I never imagined carving cocks would be my primary activity, I resolved to be as proud and honest about my work as the Wood-Working Woman was.

Years later, I would be thoughtlessly whipping out dicks of my own to wield at unwitting grocery store clerks.

These things do happen.

AN EPILOGUE, DEAR READER

People always talk about how writing a book is like having a baby. You gestate on it, spend all of this time thinking about it and growing it, and then you painstakingly push it out. When it is all said and done and you have it finished in your hands, it is beautiful and your reason for living is made clear. Or so it goes, they say. And I guess that analogy could work here for me, maybe. Writing this book was certainly a painful process of expulsion, as birthing is said to be. But the truth is, now that it is all done I can't quite be sure if it was a pregnancy or just constipation I've been experiencing. I don't know if what we have here is a newborn or a turd.

While I was writing this book over the past year, my extremely supportive mother would often ask me what exactly I was writing about. She knows what I do and what kind of blog I write. But I suppose she was hoping that my book may be a little bit more presentable, something slightly easier to share with her girlfriends than my blog has been. Alas, it is not. Not at all. So I would evade her questions every time and cringe as I thought of her (and my dad, and my grandmother, and my entire extended family) reading this. When eventually I confessed and let my mother in on the fairly obvious secret, I realized that something had to be done. Just telling my mom (and all one hundred extended family members) that my book was about my sex life and I would prefer that she not read it would not be enough. She would definitely read it. And so would my grandmother, my aunts, etc. Can you imagine if someone you love, someone you have known since they were born, someone you maybe even pushed out of your vagina, wrote a book? How could you not read that book? YOU PUSHED THAT PERSON OUT OF YOUR VAGINA. So, I get it, I do.

I decided that what had to be done was to write my family a reader's manual, so to speak. As I finished off my first draft and undertook the second, third, fourth, and fifth rewrites, I paid attention to the details. I took note of which pages I swore on, and of when I talked about my cunt and its size. I considered which chapters spoke of my sex life directly and which, if any, were slightly less vulgar. Eventually, I compiled all of this information into A Guide to Reading My Book, solely for the use of my family. I gave it to my mom and dad with a letter thanking them for all the good work they've done since my conception, for raising me and loving me without conditions (right guys? No conditions?). Doing this gave me a deep, deep sense of relief. Not only because I was experiencing the come down from the caffeine high that I had been strung out on since this book project began, but also because I felt like I finally had some context. Writing my parents a letter of explanation gave me a purpose, a way to frame this whole book thing that the writing and editing process had not done.

This does not mean that I am now sure of the value of all of this. This whole book could still be utter shit, from what I can tell. Considering that I wrote it, I have had a hard time getting a clear perspective on this one. But it is relieving to know that regardless of its calibre, I wrote a book for reasons that I feel are worth it. I did not expose my sex life, my inner monologue, and all of my not-so-secret-secrets for nothing.

It felt like a good way to end this whole thing would be to share with you my personal mail, that private letter I had written to my parents. Because we have not yet pushed the boundaries of knowing one another far enough in these pages, I want you to know not only the quantity of my urine or the size of my bodily orifices, but also just how much I love my family. I want you to know that I am a woman who carries around dildos, and someone's beloved granddaughter, a disabled person who rides a tricycle, and someone who has great sex. Identities are complex and incongruous, multi-faceted and impossible to circumnavigate. I want to be everything and to be seen as everything. Don't we all?

So let me wrap it all up by beginning it all again. Here is a letter of introduction.

Dear Mom & Dad:
A Letter of Thanks and a Guide to Reading my Book

Let me start by saying: THANK YOU. You have both done an incredible job. I am all that I am because you taught me that there is no other way to be. Mom, with your indiscriminating warmth and undaunting self-certainty, you taught me to love widely and to move through the world confidently. Dad, through your tireless efforts to call into question all forms of authority, I have learned to never be made to feel less valuable because I am different. I am quite sure that I would not have made it through the world as successfully as I have thus far if not for these tools. You have armed me well. At the end of every day, I go home loving myself because you both loved me with so much assuredness and unconditionality.

I don't know that everyone feels this way about themselves. In fact, I think most don't. And so thank you. For all of that. Now here I am, all grown up and confident enough to put all of my opinions and experiences and embarrassing anecdotes out into the world in a tangible, hold-in-your-hands, real live book. Isn't that weird? Remember just yesterday when I was a toe-sucking, bathtub-pooping, booger-eating five-year-old? How time flies.

As I am sure you have ascertained by now, considering the book is in your hands with a very descriptive back cover, this book is all about sex. "Surprise, surprise," you may think. "Our daughter is an alien. We did not produce her," you may say. "I know, I know," I respond. It may not be the most prideful thing to share with your friends and co-workers and all of our gigantic family, nor is it the easiest thing to read. This is a book about sex; my very personal ideas of and experiences with sex, to be specific.

I want to explain this all to you, lest you get the misinformed idea that your daughter is nothing but a sex-crazed weirdo, only ever thinking about orgasms and boobs and masturbating constantly. Admittedly, I do sometimes think about those things and I often masturbate. Who doesn't? But to me, sex means more than all that. To me, sex is the site where bodies may come together, and as such it is a great act to look at if you want to talk about how the world works to exclude some bodies. When we critically examine our ideas surrounding sex—what we are taught it means, what we imagine it looks like, who we think has it—we are looking at one really potent example of how a homogenous idea of "normal" is socially imposed and upheld. And the problem with "normal" is that at the end of the day, it is just a painful construct.

Wait, okay, let me step back for a second. First, let me say this: we live in a different world, you and I. Which is mostly to say that, unlike you, I am twenty-seven at a time when the internet exists. Obviously this offers a huge change from your lived reality at twenty-seven. You had babies and a mortgage. I have an iPhone and student debt. Today, with webcams, Twitter, Facebook, Instagram, blogs, etc., the personal and the private have become irreversibly blurred. The whole wide world is always in our pockets. And this means two things. One, it means that we can share anything we want to with anyone at any time. We can post selfies, write our life stories in a status update, or upload a video whenever we feel like it. And two, it means that sex has become even more omnipresent. Sex has always been a pretty pervasive beast, but now it is even more so. We can look at porn with the slide of our fingertips, we can jerk it on Chatroulette anytime we so desire. And even if we don't want to, we will find it. Sex is everywhere.

These things are not inherently bad. Sex becoming a more normalized subject of public discourse does not necessarily have to be wrong. The problem here is not the prevalence of sex. Instead, the problem is the way that sex is talked about and visualized. As sex has become more and more normalized and commodified and publicized, we see that it, too, is subject to the hegemonic idea of normal that excludes so many of us. Sex is discussed as something that only the "right" type of person, the normal type of person, the person who is white/nondisabled/cisgender/thin/young/straight has access to. Sex, we are led to believe, is not for everyone.

I hate normal. I have always hated normal, perhaps because I will never fit into it. I will never be able-bodied. I will never be straight. I will not always be thin nor young. I cannot even pretend to fit the bill. And I hate that the Rigorous Standards of Normal apply to absolutely everything, even sex. Sex, I believe, is a pretty important act. It can allow people to feel good in their bodies. It can let us feel like autonomous adults. But when sex is restricted and distorted, as it has been, it becomes inaccessible to so many people who do not or cannot conform. And not only that, but sex becomes dangerous. It becomes a symbol of power that can be taken from people without consent. It becomes a way to hurt.

So I talk about sex with all the vigor that I do because I believe that sex is important. I believe that as an act that can feel so good, it should be something that we can all have access to. I believe that as an act that has the power to hurt so bad, it should be something we talk about with more care. If we are going to see sex everywhere all of the time, I want the language with which we to talk about it, to be fair and kind. I want inclusion. I want respect.

Sex, to me, is always political. And when I talk about it, and locate myself as having it, that feels political as well. To be a queer woman with a visible disability writing about sex feels powerful and important. To write about everything, from performing terrible oral sex to having an abortion, all through the perspective of a person with a disability, is to add another voice to a conversation, a voice that is too often missing. I am not the only person doing this. I am simply mimicking some serious powerhouses doing this work. But mimicry is the ultimate form of flattery, they say, and I hope I've done a good job of it.

The version of me that I have written here is not all true. I am a shameless exaggerator, always have been. Here I wrote someone whom I sometimes am and whom I hope to be more often. I wrote a version of me who is not afraid to be unapologetically earnest. I wrote a version of me who throws herself into vulnerability with seeming abandon. I wrote a version of me who fucks and fights and loves. I wrote this version of me because to do so matters—sex-positive narratives of disability are needed.

I hope that this makes some sense to you two. I do not need you to like all of this, just not to hate it entirely, if you could. Either way, I trust that you will love me regardless of what you think of it, as you have always done. You guys may have really set yourself up for a challenge with that promise of unconditional love. I may just give in to all my impulses and go fabulously wild.

Love,
Kaleigh Annie

ACKNOWLEDGEMENTS

Birthing a baby book can't be done alone. You need all sorts of helping hands along the way providing invaluable advice, and mostly, reminding you over and over again that you are not an idiot.

I can't thank enough all the brilliant minds behind Invisible Publishing, especially Robbie for his long and thoughtful emails, and MOST ESPECIALLY Veronica Simmonds, my Book Mom. From taking my frantic phone calls on the eve of her wedding to patiently and repeatedly teaching me about Twitter. I could not have asked for a better editor/best friend. She's my best friend editor. My Bestitor. And also a huge thanks to Julia, whose grammar brain made this book coherent.

A never-ending thank you to my incredible family and friends who endured my book-related mood swings, my co-workers at Venus Envy who did the same, and my partner who talked me out of tears on more than one occasion. I am so wildly lucky to have the people in my life that I do. I pinch myself sometimes just to make sure you are all real. There are too many of you beauties to name one by one. But you know who you are. I am totally, completely, hopelessly, and endlessly in love with you.

Last but not least, thank you to YOU, you who are holding this book in your hands. Without you this whole thing would not have happened. I am forever indebted.

x&o

INVISIBLE PUBLISHING is a not-for-profit publishing company that produces contemporary works of fiction, creative non-fiction, and poetry. We publish material that's engaging, literary, current, and uniquely Canadian. We're small in scale, but we take our work, and our mission, seriously. We produce culturally relevant titles that are well written, beautifully designed, and affordable.

Invisible Publishing has been in operation for just over half a decade. Since releasing our first fiction titles in the spring of 2007, our catalogue has come to include works of graphic fiction and non-fiction, pop culture biographies, experimental poetry and prose.

Invisible Publishing continues to produce high quality literary works, we're also home to the Bibliophonic series and the Snare imprint.

If you'd like to know more please get in touch.
info@invisiblepublishing.com

Invisible Publishing
Halifax & Toronto